Super Calcium Miracle

The Calcium Citrate Malate Breakthrough

MARK ANDON, PH.D.

PRIMA HEALTH
A Division of Prima Publishing

To my family, friends, and colleagues.

Thanks for your support and patience.

Disclaimer
This book is not intended to provide medical advice and is sold with the understanding that the publisher and the author are not liable for the misconception or misuse of information provided. The author and Prima Publishing shall have neither liability nor responsibility to any person or entity with respect to any loss, damage, or injury caused or alleged to be caused directly or indirectly by the information contained in this book or the use of any products mentioned. Readers should not use any of the products discussed in this book without the advice of a medical professional.

The production of this work was not underwritten in any way by the pharmaceutical companies whose products are mentioned.

Library of Congress Cataloging-in-Publication Data

Andon, Mark.
Super calcium miracle : the calcium citrate malate breakthrough / Mark Andon.
p. cm.
Includes bibliographical references and index.
ISBN 0-7615-1456-2
1. Calcium citrate malate—Therapeutic use. 2. Osteoporosis—Chemotherapy. I. Title.
RC931.073A536 1998
616.7′16—dc21 98-25969
CIP

98 99 00 01 02 HH 10 9 8 7 6 5 4 3 2 1
Printed in the United States of America

CONTENTS

INTRODUCTION

Of all the minerals in your body, calcium is present in the highest amount. In fact, the amount of calcium you possess just about equals all the other minerals put together. Not surprisingly, your body's need for calcium is also the highest of any mineral or vitamin. Calcium plays a central role in your body's most basic life functions, such as sperm motility, egg fertilization, hormone action, and cell reproduction. The structural integrity of your bones and teeth depends on calcium. In addition, calcium is vital to many biochemical processes, including muscle contraction, nerve conduction, and the control of enzyme reactions.

Due to calcium's critical importance in virtually every cell, your body controls calcium levels more tightly than those of any other nutrient. If your calcium intake is too low to meet metabolic demands, your body's set of highly regulated control mechanisms, specifically designed to pull calcium out of your bones, goes to work. This action keeps your blood calcium concentration at the proper level and your cells functioning normally. In other words, the rest of your body takes "calcium priority" over your skeleton.

Ideally, your calcium intake should be high enough so that your body doesn't have to choose between your bones and other body systems. However, the calcium intake of most people falls well short of the right amount. Only one out of every 10 women, and three out of every 10 men, consume the recommended level of calcium. This fact may seem hard to believe given the obvious abundance and availability of food in America. We are usually concerned with eating too much, not too little. However, the reverse is true of calcium. The link between our low calcium intake and its negative effect on health has been recognized by several public health organizations, including the Department of Health and Human Services, the National Institutes of Health, and the National Research Council. The ultimate impact of inadequate calcium intake is reduced building of bone during growth and accelerated loss of bone during aging. Either of these circumstances places you at increased risk for osteoporosis.

Osteoporosis, or fragile bone disease, is the most common skeletal disorder in the world. In the United States alone, it affects 25 million people and accounts for 1.5 million new fractures per year. Although every part of the skeleton becomes weak and more prone to injury with this disorder, the majority of fractures occur in the spine and hip. Sixty percent of women ages 70 years or older have at least one osteoporotic compression fracture in the spine. Many women will suffer from multiple compression fractures and completely collapsed vertebrae. These vertebral fractures lead to pain, loss of self-esteem, reduced ability to carry out daily activities, and a decrease in height that can total as much as six to eight inches. In very severe cases the spine compresses so much that the only thing preventing further loss in height is the rib cage resting on top of the pelvic bones.

Although vertebral fractures are the most common, hip fractures are the most devastating aspect of osteoporosis. A woman's risk of hip fracture is slightly greater than her *combined* risk of developing breast, uterine, and ovarian cancers. Moreover, because hip fractures have a high mortality rate associated with them, the number of women dying each year from osteoporosis equals the deaths attributed to breast cancer. Men are not immune to osteoporosis or its consequences, either. They have a fracture risk two to four times lower than a woman's, but their death rate following a hip fracture is twice as great. The risk of hip fracture in a man is the same as his risk of developing prostate cancer.

Osteoporosis has been called the "silent thief" because bone loss occurs gradually over time, without obvious signs or symptoms. Like every other organ system in the body, bone is a living tissue, constantly turning over and renewing itself. As older bone tissue is broken down, new bone tissue is made to replace it. Bone loss occurs when the balance between bone synthesis and breakdown is upset. Although a number of lifestyle factors can upset this balance, calcium is recognized as the most important nutritional factor. There isn't any blood test you can take to tell if you're consuming enough calcium. Your body maintains a steady blood level by using the calcium you eat or by taking calcium out of your bones. In America today, essentially 100% of women and 90%–95% of men over the age of 50 fail to consume the optimal level of dietary calcium. Younger women and teenage girls are also high-risk groups, with over 90% consuming sub-optimal amounts. The low calcium intake in these younger females is of great concern because bones reach their peak calcium content at about 20 years of age and bone loss ensues soon afterward (well before menopause).

Recognition of the importance of calcium during all phases of the life cycle has rapidly evolved during the last 10 to 15 years. Some of the most significant findings in this research arena have been generated using a special calcium source called CCM *(calcium citrate malate)*. Developed by the Procter & Gamble Company, CCM is a premier source of calcium that has repeatedly produced superior results. Its safety and effectiveness are backed by studies funded through the National Institutes of Health and the United States Department of Agriculture.

CCM has been evaluated at leading universities and medical centers throughout the country. A number of landmark studies in the field of calcium nutrition and bone health have utilized CCM and have played an integral part in defining the optimal level of calcium intake. These important findings have been published in our country's most prestigious scientific journals of medicine and nutrition. Despite the rich scientific history and sterling performance record of CCM, this supplement is not very well-known in the health care community or by consumers. As such, I hope this book will heighten public awareness of the importance of calcium and serve as a useful educational guide regarding the remarkable results obtained by the men, women, and children who have taken CCM.

CHAPTER ONE

How Much Calcium Do I Need?

- Why You Should Double Your Calcium Intake Now
- Humans Evolved As High-Calcium Consumers
- Calcium Intake—Our National Deficit
- Calcium Citrate Malate—A Better Way to Improve Calcium Intake
- Recommendations for Optimal Calcium Intake

Ninety-nine percent of the body's calcium resides in the skeleton where it functions as the basic building block of bone. The other 1% is distributed throughout the body and serves a multitude of purposes such as regulating muscles, nerves, enzymes, and communication systems within all cells.[1] Because calcium is so vital to these *ex skeletal* (outside the skeleton) functions, your body always takes care of them first. Your bones play second fiddle to the rest of the body when it comes to meeting calcium requirements. This is why you can't detect a calcium deficiency until it's too late. Even if your calcium intake is very low, your body adapts to keep cells outside the skeleton functioning like they should.

However, you pay a price for having this safeguard mechanism. Although everything else is functioning normally, if you don't get enough calcium when you're young, you won't build a strong skeleton during your formative years. Similarly, if your calcium intake falls short as an adult, your body weakens your skeleton by robbing it of calcium for use in other cellular functions throughout your body. For this reason, the amount of calcium you need for total health (both cellular functions and skeletal demands) is the amount that optimizes bone strength.

Your optimal calcium intake varies throughout your life cycle according to your age and physiological condition. For example, children going through the rapid growth spurt of puberty need more calcium because their skeletons are growing very fast. Older individuals need more calcium because their ability to retain the calcium in their bones is diminished. In this chapter you will learn why humans are metabolically adapted to thrive on a high-calcium diet. You'll also learn why our current diets fall well short of these levels and discover what scientists and doctors are saying about the latest recommendations for optimal calcium intake.

Why You Should Double Your Calcium Intake Now

Most people have no idea how much calcium they usually consume or how much they should be consuming. Unfortunately, this puts them at a great disadvantage for reducing their risk of developing osteoporosis, or fragile bone disease. Osteoporosis accounts for 1.5 million fractures and $14 billion in medical expenses per year in the United States alone.[2] Mortality after a hip fracture is estimated to be 24% during the first year following the fracture. In addition, about 50% of all hip fracture survivors who were able to walk independently *before* the fracture need assistance *after* the fracture, and about one-third may lose their independence altogether.[3] That's why older people are afraid of falling. It's not the fall itself that scares them; rather, it's that they know someone, or know *of* someone, who fell, broke a hip, and either died or had to be institutionalized as a result.

Low calcium intake is a major risk factor for developing osteoporosis. More importantly, our calcium intake is something we can all change to reduce our chances of falling prey to this degenerative disorder. Genetics play a big role in this disease, but you can't change your genes. Exercising on a regular basis helps guard against osteoporosis, but many people lack the self-discipline to stick with an exercise program. Although it's impossible to ignore our genetic makeup and it may *seem* impossible to undertake an exercise program, the nutritional factor is much easier for us to control. We all have to eat and it's something we enjoy doing. Making simple, informed choices about the foods, drinks, and supplements we consume can make all the difference in the world when it comes to boosting our calcium intake.

The typical postmenopausal woman in the United States currently consumes about 600 mg of calcium per day.[4] This figure falls well below the recommended 1,200-mg level recently set by the National Academy of Sciences, and even further below the 1,500-mg level set by the National Institutes of Health Consensus Conference on Optimal Calcium Intake (see Figure 1-1).[1,5] Part

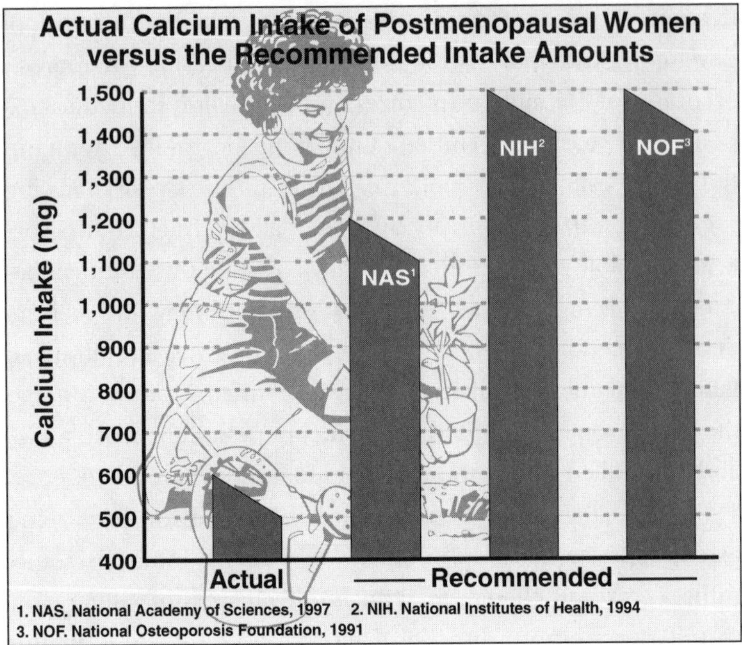

Figure 1-1

of the problem is that the typical woman doesn't realize she needs to at least *double* her calcium intake. First of all, no one thinks they're typical. In fact, a recent national survey found that 50% of women believe their calcium intake is just about right.[4] Second, you can't *feel* a calcium deficiency. There are no obvious signs or symptoms to tell you that your body is craving more calcium. That's the insidious nature of the bone-loss process.

Humans Evolved As High-Calcium Consumers

To understand our need for calcium today, we must understand calcium's role in the development of our species. As the process of evolution and adaptation marched steadily forward in time, it was in response to environmental demands. If elements critical to our survival were in abundant supply and were easy to obtain, then our bodies didn't need to make any special adaptations for our biological demands to be met. If the availability of critical elements changed very slowly over time, then our bodies' process of adaptation could keep step and could provide solutions to the changing environment. On the other hand, if a critical element were to be suddenly removed from our environment or greatly reduced in availability, then our physiological adaptations could not keep pace and the health of our species would be compromised. As you will see, the low amounts of calcium in our self-selected diets of today are a clear departure from the high-calcium environment that was present throughout our evolutionary journey. Simply put, we are asking too much from our genetic makeup when we expect our bodies to successfully deal with the greatly reduced amounts of calcium that have recently occurred in our diet as a result of cultural and technological changes.

What were the amounts of calcium available to living creatures during our slow, but continuous, progression from single-celled organisms to modern-day humans? To begin with, calcium is readily found in large amounts throughout our natural environment. It is the fifth most abundant mineral in both the earth's crust and in seawater.[6] Calcium is also the fifth most abundant element in the human body, as well as its most abundant mineral. It is preceded only by the elements hydrogen, oxygen, carbon, and nitrogen. Hydrogen and oxygen are present in such large amounts due to the high water content in our bodies (70% of the body's weight is water). Carbon is the basic component of all the organic matter we are made of, and nitrogen is the distinguishing building block of protein.

Life on earth emerged and evolved in a calcium-rich environment. Information about the calcium supply that existed at a much later period in the evolutionary timescale—from a mere 200 million years ago up to the present day—was pieced together by researchers from Emory and Wayne State Universities, from studying anthropology, primate evolution, and nutrition.[7] As they explain, early small mammals made their inconspicuous appearance about 200 million years ago. These early mammals were primarily insect eaters. Because the exoskeleton of insects is very rich in calcium, the diet of these early mammals was also very rich in calcium. Thus, the forerunners of our primate ancestors evolved with a high calcium intake.

You can't feel *a calcium deficiency. There are no obvious signs or symptoms to tell you that your body is craving more calcium.*

Shortly after the mass extinction of the dinosaurs, about 60 million years ago, the fossil record reveals the first appearance of nonhuman primates—our closest relatives. Like their ancestors, early primates subsisted to a large extent on an insect-based diet that was high in calcium. However, as time passed and evolution continued, the primate diet became more and more varied. Besides insects, it included more fruits, leaves, seeds, and other plant material. Today's nonhuman primates have diets similar to this. Our closest primate relative, the chimpanzee, has a genetic composition that is 98%–99% identical to ours. The chimpanzee's diet in the wild is composed of many foods, including meat, leaves, insects, fruits, seeds, and so forth. Analysis of the naturally occurring diet of the chimpanzee shows that it contains approximately four times as much calcium as our human diet, on a gram for gram basis.

Earliest Homo sapiens (literally, "thinking man") are believed to have appeared sometime between 100,000 years and 1.5 million years ago on the African continent. Anatomically, modern humans date back about 40,000 or 45,000 years ago. From a genetic standpoint, these late-stone-age men and women are essentially the same as your next-door neighbor, having the same physiology, biochemistry, and nutritional needs.

Modern human beings aggressively spread into Europe, Asia, and eventually North America via the Bering Straits, and then southward to the rest of the Americas. At this point in time, possibly as early as 90,000 years ago or as late as 20,000 years ago, we were still interacting with our food environment in a natural way. We had become more efficient at hunting and ate considerable quantities of wild game, but we relied heavily on wild plants for most of our caloric intake. Up to this point, our physical and biochemical adaptations had kept pace with our cultural and technological evolution. The process had been slow and gradual, but a major change was about to occur that would drastically alter the way we lived. Along with this change would come fateful alterations in our food supply of calcium and other nutrients.

Man invented agriculture about 10,000 years ago, and we began to exert control over our food environment like never before. The raising of livestock and the cultivation of crops became widespread. The variety in our diet decreased as we shifted from consuming a wide range of wild plants to relying on cultivated grains. Grains, especially cultivated grains, contain much less calcium than wild plants do. Furthermore, we learned to select and develop crop characteristics to increase yields. However, the characteristics we selected mainly increased the caloric and starch content of the grains at the expense of protein, vitamins, and minerals. This had a double negative impact on our calcium intake. Cultivated grains contain less calcium than their wild counterparts, and we didn't need to eat as much of the cultivated grain in order to meet our caloric needs.

Another major dietary difference between stone-age man and your typical American suburbanite is the abundance of milk as the main source of calcium in the present-day diet. Until the domestication of animals, no primate, be it Homo sapiens or one of our nonhuman primate relatives, ever consumed milk other than mother's milk during infancy and early childhood. Even today, most of the world's populations do not practice the consumption of milk obtained from other species. Lactose (milk sugar) intolerance is prevalent in most areas of the world—in Asia, Africa, the Indian subcontinent, the Near East, the Mediterranean, the Pacific Islands, and Latin America.[1,8] It even occurs in indigenous populations of North America, among various Native American tribes. In addition, the practice of drinking milk from domesticated animals is a relatively recent event that began only 2,000 years ago. Thus, in the grand scheme of evolution, the use of milk is a very new, relatively untested, and not widely practiced strategy for meeting nutritional calcium needs.

The recent shift from a diet rich in calcium to our current low-calcium diet is a challenge to our biochemistry. If you compress the unbroken evolutionary timescale from the first appearance of mammals to the present into a single 24-hour day, then our exposure to this new low-calcium diet has existed for only four seconds. From a cultural and technological standpoint, we have greatly outpaced our physical and biochemical ability to adapt.

The relatively high dietary calcium intake during most of our evolution provides strong justification for incorporating greater amounts of calcium in our present-day diet. However, much of this hypothesis is based on educated guesswork. We can't actually gauge the diets our ancestors adapted to through the millennia, which is the diet we are presumably best suited to thrive on. However, there are things we can directly measure today that support the notion that man evolved on a high-calcium diet. This evidence gives us a good sense of our nutritional needs in the distant past and a way to better understand our present and future nutritional needs.

A study of howler and spider monkeys living in Guatemala shows that the average calcium content of their food supply contains 907 mg of calcium per 1,000 calories.[9] Recent data from the U.S. Department of Agriculture reveals that the average adult person consumes only 350–400 mg of calcium per 1,000 calories.[4] Furthermore, the caloric expenditure of animals in the wild is greater than that of humans living a modern sedentary lifestyle. Thus, our nonhuman primate counterparts consume relatively greater amounts of foods that are higher in calcium content than we do.

Perhaps the most relevant information concerning the diet that humans ate prior to the agricultural revolution comes from studies of hunter-gatherer groups. These societies generally reflect the lifestyle and dietary practices that existed among early hominids. These practices date back as far as 4 million years ago and have continued up to modern times, just prior to the advent of agricultural societies. Although they are few and far between, a number of these groups still exist today. They have been the topic of scholarly investigations, which include surveys of the amount and nutrient content of their foods.[10]

The dietary characteristics of modern-day hunter-gatherer groups include a reliance on wild game and the consumption of a wide range of wild vegetable foods, including roots, tubers, fruits, beans, nuts, and flowers. The calcium density of many of these wild plants is extremely high compared to that of our modern cultivated crops. For example, a survey of edible wild plants shows that they contain an average of 1.3 mg of calcium per gram.[7] Compare this value to milk, which contains 1.2 mg of calcium per gram. In addition, many of these plants contain three to four times the amount of calcium as milk does, on a per gram basis. Thus, the potential is high for a hunter-gatherer to have a diet abundant in calcium. Using the average calcium content of wild plant foods and assuming that hunter-gatherers obtained 35% of their total calories from wild game (which is much lower in calcium than plants, only 0.14 mg of calcium per gram), the daily calcium intake for humans prior to the age of agriculture is estimated to have been 1,800 mg. If they obtained a larger proportion of their total calories from non-meat sources, say 80%, then their calcium intake is estimated to have been about 2,100 mg.[10]

Clearly, modern-day humans have made a huge departure from our evolutionary beginnings as high-calcium consumers. How we are adapting to this low-calcium diet, and at what cost to society, is an experiment-in-progress. Obviously, we're not going to turn the clock back to preagricultural days. However, there are other strategies and adaptations we can make to provide a diet that more closely mimics the intake we are genetically designed for. In terms of calcium, these approaches include the intelligent selection of high-calcium foods, including the use of calcium-fortified foods and beverages and supplementation of the diet.

Bones are like a savings account at the bank. Instead of depositing money, you add calcium to your bone bank account. Carrying this analogy a step further, we all know that when it comes to planning for retirement, the sooner you start saving and the more you save, the better off you will be.

Calcium Intake—Our National Deficit

The value of calcium and the need to boost intakes are not limited to postmenopausal women. There is a lifelong need to optimize calcium intake to help ensure a strong skeleton. Bones are like a savings account at the bank. Instead of depositing money, you add calcium to your bone bank account.

Carrying this analogy a step further, we all know that when it comes to planning for retirement, the sooner you start saving and the more you save, the better off you will be. The same applies for your calcium bank account. Making deposits when you're young and continuing to make them on a regular basis will pay big dividends in the future. Although research shows it's never too late for calcium to have a positive impact on bone health (even women in their eighties have benefited), it's also never too early to begin laying the foundation for bone health. Sadly, as a nation, we are becoming very poor investors in our calcium bank accounts. Average calcium intake is 8% lower now than it was in the early 1970s.[4,11]

As the large baby boom population grows older and starts entering the time of life when there is high risk for developing osteoporosis, a tidal wave of osteoporotic fractures is predicted to occur.

If you combine our low-calcium diet with our continued advance in life expectancy, a very disturbing picture develops. Remember, bone loss in adulthood is a slow, gradual process. Thus, the longer you live, the greater your chance for developing osteoporosis. We *are* living longer. Average life expectancy has increased from about 45 to 50 years of age at the turn of the century to our present 73 to 80 years.[12]. However, we are now even less vigilant about consuming the recommended levels of calcium that would reduce the risk of osteoporosis. Furthermore, many children are consuming less than optimal amounts of calcium during the bone-building years. This leads to them becoming adults with less calcium reserves stored in their bones. The situation is a double jeopardy for bone health—children building less bone and adults losing more bone. If this trend is not reversed, it may have extreme consequences for our medical care system. As the large baby boom population grows older and starts entering the time of life when there is high risk for developing osteoporosis, a tidal wave of osteoporotic fractures is predicted to occur. By 2040, the year the average baby boomer will be 85 years old, the estimated number of hip fractures could be as high as 840,000 per year.[12] Extrapolating the current costs of medical care for hip and all other osteoporotic fractures, this equates to a total cost to our medical care system of $47 billion (in 1998 dollars). Factoring in a relatively modest rate of inflation for medical care, of 3% per year, the total bill for osteoporosis could reach $163 billion by 2040.

Typical Calcium Intakes Fall Short

Because nationwide statistics on calcium intake in the United States have been collected since the 1970s, we can track the progress of various age groups for bolstering calcium intake.[4,11] Although all age groups fall short of the recommended intakes, children in particular have experienced a dramatic drop in their calcium intake. Compared to 25 years ago, children ages 5 and younger consume 8% less calcium, those ages 6 to 11 years get 15%–20% less, and calcium consumption by teenagers is down 7%–15%. Adult men have stayed about the same. The only group that has made some progress is adult females. Their average calcium intake has increased about 30 mg, or 5%, compared to the early 1970s. However, adult females still lag far behind the other age and sex groups for total calcium intake. As a group, teenage boys are the highest calcium consumers. They are followed in descending order by preadolescent boys, adult men, preadolescent girls, and young children (toddlers). Adult women and teenage girls come in at last place in the calcium race—yet many experts in the calcium nutrition field recognize that teenage girls and older adult women have the greatest needs for calcium. Unfortunately, however, many women believe they're getting plenty of calcium. A recent survey by the U.S. Department of Agriculture found that 50% of adult women believe their current calcium intake is at the right level.[4] But the reality is that very few women are getting the recommended amount of calcium. For women ages 51 years or older:

- Essentially 100% consume less than the recommended amount of calcium.
- 80% consume less than two-thirds the recommended amount of calcium.
- 50% consume less than one-half the recommended amount of calcium.
- 30% consume less than one-third the recommended amount of calcium.

Men are equally, if not more, confused about their calcium intake. The U.S. Department of Agriculture survey found that 60% thought their calcium intake was at the right level. However, men don't do much better than women. For men ages 51 years or older:

- 90%–95% consume less than the recommended amount of calcium.
- 60% consume less than two-thirds the recommended amount of calcium.
- 40% consume less than one-half the recommended amount of calcium.
- 15% consume less than one-third the recommended amount of calcium.

Even teenage boys, the group with the greatest calcium intake, fall short of the recommended amount of calcium. About seven out of 10 teenage boys get less than the recommended amount of calcium, and four out of every 10 are consuming less than one-half the recommended amount. Teenage girls are even worse, with about 90%–95% getting less than the recommended amount.

Milk Isn't the Answer

When new research about the benefits of obtaining more calcium is published, the message that often gets conveyed to the consumer is "drink more milk." This is the case even when milk is not the source of the calcium used in the research. In fact, the type of research with the highest degree of scientific merit can't use milk because milk has no placebo. You can't do a double-blind, placebo-controlled, randomized trial without a placebo. Nevertheless, the media routinely chooses to single out milk as the preferred approach for consuming more calcium.

Compared to 25 years ago, children ages 5 and younger consume 8% less calcium, those ages 6 to 11 years get 15%–20% less, and calcium consumption by teenagers is down 7%–15%.

Why has the "drink more milk" approach been taken to communicate the benefits of calcium, and what has been the outcome? In the United States, milk is viewed as the gold standard of calcium-rich foods. The dairy industry has been active for many years in promoting milk through advertising and educational efforts. Paralleling the dairy industry's efforts, the U.S. Department of Agriculture's system for conveying nutrition information has emphasized milk (dairy products). Milk has been established as a staple food in the U.S. agricultural and food supply system—first, as a member of the now outdated "four food groups" and, more recently, as one of the groups in the "Food Guide Pyramid." As a dietary staple and a commodity food item, it's more comfortable for health authorities to recommend milk because the recommendation doesn't benefit any one particular company or brand of product. In addition, due to the general lack of other calcium-rich food products in the typical person's diet, milk remains a primary source of calcium.

What has been the result of communicating positive health news about calcium in terms of recommending more milk consumption? Milk intake has been flat or declining for the past two decades. An exception to this trend has occurred during the last two years or so, with milk intake up slightly. Credit for this increase goes to the dairy industry's effort to expand the variety of milk products (such as flavored milks) and to the multimillion-dollar advertising campaigns "Got milk?" and the "milk mustache." So what's wrong with milk? Why is the dairy industry saying "Got milk?" but the consumer is saying "not milk"? There's nothing wrong with milk, per se. It's a fine food and a very rich source of calcium for those who like it. It's just that people are already drinking as much as they're going to. Milk is already widely consumed, especially among children. However, a tremendous change in milk-consuming habits would be needed in order to meet the recommended optimal calcium intake goals. Let's look at the numbers.[4]

On any given day, 85% of kids, ages 1 to 5 years old, drink some amount of milk. The numbers drop to 75%–80% for kids 6 to 11 years old, 50%–60% for teenagers, and level off at about 50% for adults. Milk is by far our predominant dairy food. For example, only 4% of the population consumes yogurt on any given day. Milk-based desserts such as ice cream are higher, at 18%, and cheese comes in a strong second to milk, at 32%.

As far as the quantity of milk consumption goes, young kids are the stars again. Kids ages 1 to 2 years consume a little over 1.5 cups per day. For girls, this consumption drops to slightly more than one cup by the time they're in grade school, continues to drop during the teen years to less than a cup, and levels off in adult females at about one-half cup per day. For males, the pattern is much the same, except they maintain a higher level of consumption for a longer period of time. The fall-off in milk consumption for boys is typically seen around the legal drinking age. Milk consumption goes down and levels off in adult males, to about three-quarters of a cup per day.

The difference in timing between the sexes for the drop in milk consumption is probably related to psychosocial factors. Boys may view milk as a food that helps make them strong. In contrast, girls are concerned with the fat and caloric content of milk and may view it as a food for babies and young children. In addition, kids don't observe their parents drinking milk. This undoubtedly has an impact on their behavior as they mature.

Whole milk (3.3%–3.5% milk fat) accounts for about one-third of the total milk consumed, 2% milk represents nearly one-half of the total, and skim milk (no fat) makes up the balance at about 20% of the total. A couple of milk myths worth mentioning involve the fat and calcium content in milk. Many people believe that calcium is removed when the fat content of milk is lowered. However, the opposite actually occurs (see Table 1-1 for the composition of milk products). The lower the fat content, the more calcium there is in the milk.[13] That's because calcium is in the water portion of milk, not the fat portion. Another myth is that 2% milk is low in fat; the reality, however, is that about 35% of the calories in 2% milk are from fat. In contrast, a lot of people think that buttermilk is high in fat because it contains butter. In fact, the opposite is true; buttermilk is essentially what's left over after the butterfat has been removed, and it is actually lower in fat content than 2% milk. Calorie- and fat-wise, whole chocolate milk is the

Table 1-1 Milk Composition*

Milk Type	*Calories*	*Fat (g)*	*% Fat Calories*	*Sugar (g)*	*Protein (g)*	*Calcium (mg)*
Whole	150	8.1	49	11	8	291
2%	121	4.7	35	12	8	297
Skim	86	0.4	5	12	8	302
Buttermilk	99	2.2	20	12	8	285
Chocolate	208	8.5	27	26	8	280
Chocolate 2%	179	5.0	25	26	8	284

** based on an 8-ounce serving*

poorest selection. It has the most fat, the most calories, and the least calcium.

The average postmenopausal woman would need to quintuple her milk intake to increase her current inadequate calcium intake to the recommended level. This shows the ineffectiveness of prior efforts to make milk consumption a more palatable option for increasing calcium consumption. Thus, while I favor continued efforts to promote greater milk intake, the overemphasis on milk, which has occurred in the past, is not the answer. This is the case for any single food. No one product can do it alone, because eating behaviors and food patterns are remarkably difficult to change. If a person starts drinking more milk, that generally means they need to stop drinking something else. Whatever that something else is, chances are that most people don't want to give it up.

A more realistic adjunct approach is to find appropriate foods and beverages to fortify. An appropriate food would be one to which calcium can be added without negatively impacting its taste or appearance. The food or beverage would also need to have a high enough frequency of consumption, at least by certain segments of the population, so that a real impact on calcium intake could be made. Orange juice and juice drinks with calcium are good examples of this. Both are well liked, widely consumed, and consumed with enough frequency to impact millions of people. A bad example would be something like caviar. Even if you like it, how often can you eat it?

The average postmenopausal woman would need to quintuple her milk intake to increase her current inadequate calcium intake to the recommended level.

Of course, the other viable approach is supplementation, which requires a behavioral change but not a change in food patterns. Although a lot of calcium supplements are sold in this country, many of the bottles end up sitting on top of the refrigerator gathering dust. If you're going to use this approach, it's not enough to just buy the supplements. You need to take them on a daily basis. In addition, as you will discover in subsequent chapters, the effectiveness of the particular calcium source used in supplements can vary. Check the labels!

Calcium carbonate is the most common source of calcium used in the vast majority of both brand name and generic calcium supplements. It's also used in some antacid tablets, which can be taken to supply calcium. Be sure to read the label carefully on antacid products if you're using them to increase your calcium intake. Not all of them contain calcium carbonate as part of the active ingredients to neutralize stomach acid.

Lack of Other Calcium-Rich Foods

Another reason for our national deficit in calcium intake is the general lack of other calcium-rich foods in the average diet. Once you count dairy products and calcium-fortified foods and beverages, the list gets pretty short. Although you may see alternative suggestions for calcium-containing foods in the popular press, these are usually of little practical importance. For example, despite the fact that only 5% of the calcium from spinach is absorbed, it still gets recommended as a way to boost calcium intake.[14] It's not that spinach isn't a fine food; it's a wonderful food but a lousy source of calcium. Other vegetables, such as broccoli and brussels sprouts, supply calcium that's very well-absorbed—in fact, their absorption is better than is the calcium from milk.[15] The problem is they are relatively low in calcium content. You need to eat five servings of broccoli or eight servings of brussels sprouts to get the same amount of absorbed calcium as a cup of milk. Two alternative sources of calcium that sometimes get recommended because they are relatively high in calcium content are canned fish (with the bones included) and tofu (which uses a calcium salt treatment to coagulate the soybean proteins into a curd). The obvious problem with these foods is that very few people want to eat them. The take-away message is simple. Unless you're a big milk drinker (six to eight times the average consumption), you had better be using calcium-fortified foods or supplements if you want to hit the optimal calcium intake level on a daily basis.

Calcium Citrate Malate— A Better Way to Improve Calcium Intake

Given our national calcium deficit, scientists have been greatly encouraged by the test results of a new form of calcium—calcium citrate malate (CCM). As I mentioned earlier, a better approach to improving calcium intake than increasing the amount of milk you drink would be to fortify foods you already consume or to take supplements. Research has shown that beverages fortified with CCM and supplements containing CCM can improve not only calcium absorption but also skeletal health throughout the human life cycle.

CCM is composed of calcium in combination with two organic acids, citric acid and malic acid. They are commonly called "fruit acids" because of their natural abundance in virtually all fruits. Citric acid is found in oranges, grapefruits, and strawberries, and malic acid is predominantly in apples, pears, and many berries. Citric and malic acids also occur naturally in the human body; they are made during the energy production cycle of the cell.

Interestingly, the original research on CCM in the early to mid-1980s had nothing to do with its nutritional benefits but, rather, exclusively focused on finding a palatable way to increase the calcium content of beverages. At that point in time, no one imagined the groundbreaking discoveries that would result from work on CCM in the fields of nutrition and bone health science. In the early developmental work, scientists discovered that CCM possessed two important attributes that made it particularly useful in fortifying beverages. Because its calcium was combined with fruit acids, CCM had outstanding solubility characteristics and was highly compatible with a variety of fruit flavors. Normally, adding calcium to a beverage imparts a chalky off-flavor. In addition, most calcium sources are not soluble enough to permit high levels of calcium to dissolve in a beverage. CCM's combination of taste compatibility and solubility permitted the development of calcium-fortified beverages with as much calcium as milk.

The next critical step was the decision to measure CCM's calcium absorption performance. To appreciate the significance of this, you must keep in mind the environment in which food, beverage, and/or supplement companies operate. Manufacturers are not required to measure how much of the calcium in their products can be absorbed into the human body. All they have to do is verify the total amount of calcium that is claimed on the label. Thus, very few products have been evaluated for their calcium absorption. However, to truly be useful to our bodies, the calcium needs to be *absorbed*. Humans are quite inefficient at utilizing calcium and there is a very wide range of calcium absorption from various foods.

The initial assessment of calcium absorption from CCM compared it to milk and calcium carbonate. Milk and dairy products account for approximately 75% of the total food calcium consumed in the United States, and calcium carbonate is the main form of calcium used in supplement pills. Calcium absorption from CCM was found to be significantly *greater* than from either milk or calcium carbonate![15–25] This surprising discovery provided the impetus for a long string of additional studies, which have clearly established CCM as one of the most thoroughly tested calcium sources in the world. Several studies demonstrated that calcium absorption from CCM is 40% greater than other sources of calcium. Long-term studies involving CCM have shown significant bone building in children and postmenopausal women and a reduction in fractures in both older men and women.[26–37] No other calcium source can claim this combination of clinically proven benefits.

Where Can I Get CCM?

CCM is currently available in a number of calcium-fortified beverages and in a calcium supplement form. In the future, CCM may appear in more products as the public becomes aware of its remarkable characteristics. The following beverages contain CCM: Sunny Delight with Calcium, Tropicana Pure Premium Orange Juice with Calcium and Extra Vitamin C, Tropicana Bursters, and certain versions of Beech-Nut brand baby and toddler juices. CCM is identified in these beverage products using the name "FruitCal." A FruitCal logo appears on the product packages, but it isn't very large, so check the labels carefully.

CCM also comes in several supplement forms and is identified by the name "Calcium Citrate Malate." At present, you can't get them at a regular drug or grocery store; however, they are sold exclusively at GNC stores under the name Calcimate.

Although these products use different names, they all contain CCM. Similarly, if you read about CCM in the newspaper, a magazine, or health newsletter, it may be identified as CCM, calcium citrate malate, and/or FruitCal. Furthermore, the companies that use CCM in their products may interchangeably call it calcium citrate malate, CCM, and/or FruitCal in their product information literature.

Recommendations for Optimal Calcium Intake

A great deal of time and energy has been spent by nutrition and medical scientists to arrive at a set of calcium intake recommendations that individuals can use as a yardstick to measure whether they are getting enough calcium. Some of the best minds in the calcium research field have worked together to answer the question "How much calcium do I need?" As a result, guidelines have been established by three important groups—the National Institutes of Health, the National Osteoporosis Foundation, and the National Academy of Sciences. Although much of the same information has been used by each of these groups to determine intake guidelines, the recommendations don't always match up. In fact, some of the recommendations differ greatly, by as much as 50% or more. One thing calcium researchers consistently agree on is that people should be consuming more calcium than they are now. As shown in Figure 1-2, the current recommendations for calcium intake fall within the following ranges:

Preadolescent children—800–1,200 mg

Adolescents and young adults—1,200–1,500 mg

Adults—1,000 mg

Adults ages 50 or older—1,000–1,500 mg

The National Institutes Of Health

The National Institutes of Health (NIH) comprise the largest biomedical research organization in the country. In 1994, the

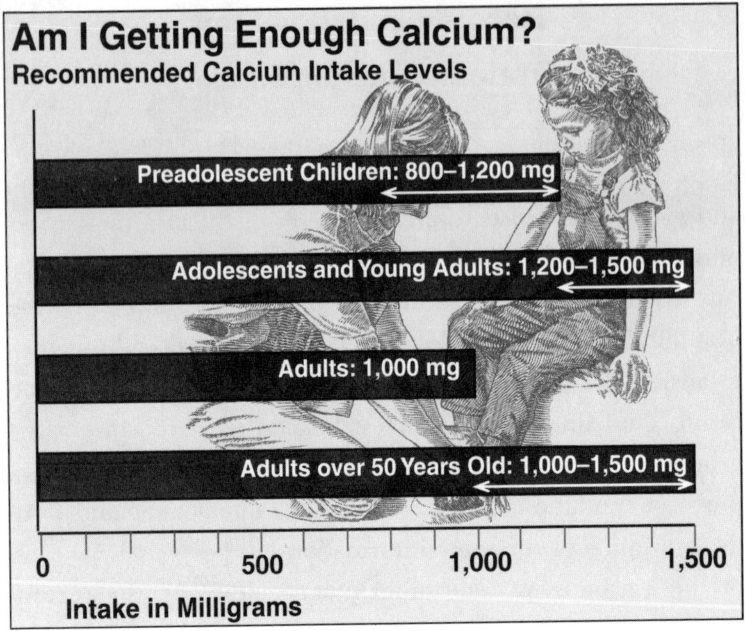

Figure 1-2

NIH called together some of greatest minds in the calcium research field to develop a set of guidelines for Optimal Calcium Intake.[5] The word *optimal* is very important. Although we can survive on relatively little calcium, an optimal intake allows us to best increase our chances of having good skeletal health all our lives and to reduce our risk of developing osteoporosis. The blue-ribbon panel that gathered in June 1994 at the NIH in Bethesda, Maryland, defined optimal calcium intake in the following way: First, for children, optimal calcium intake is the amount that allows them to maximize the building of bone during their growth and development years. This is a critical concept because 90% to 95% of the total bone mass you will ever have is built by the time you reach your late teens.[38] Second, optimal calcium intake for adults is the amount that allows you to maintain the bone mass you built as a child and as an adolescent and to minimize the loss of bone that occurs in your later years. Keep in mind that building bone is not like pouring concrete. Our whole skeleton is a living tissue that constantly turns over and is renewed. This process, known as "bone remodeling," requires a balance between the breakdown of old bone tissue and the buildup of new bone tissue. As we age, we lose the ability to keep this balance in check. More calcium helps to restore the balance and keep our bones strong. The optimal calcium intakes defined by the NIH are:

From birth to 6 months of age—400 mg

From 6 months to 1 year—600 mg

Ages 1 to 5 years—800 mg

Ages 6 to 10 years—1,200 mg

Ages 11 to 24 years—1,200 to 1,500 mg

Men ages 25 to 65 years—1,000 mg

Adult women up to menopause—1,000 mg

Postmenopausal women—1,500 mg

Men ages 65 years or older—1,500 mg

The National Osteoporosis Foundation

The National Osteoporosis Foundation (NOF) is an advocacy group based in Washington, D.C., that fights for increased funding to discover ways of preventing and treating osteoporosis.

They also make available high quality educational materials on osteoporosis to physicians and consumers, sponsor osteoporosis education conferences, and directly support osteoporosis research with their own funding. In 1991, the NOF made their own recommendations on calcium intakes.[39] The NOF's philosophy was much the same as that of the NIH—that is, a preventive approach to osteoporosis that includes a calcium intake high enough to ensure maximal bone building in children and minimal bone loss in adults. The calcium intake recommendations from the NOF are:

Ages 1 to 24 years—1,200 mg

For men over age 24—1,000 mg

For women over age 24 up to menopause—1,000 mg

For women after menopause—1,500 mg

The National Academy of Sciences

The most recent recommendations for calcium intake were made by the Food and Nutrition Board in 1997.[1] The Food and Nutrition Board is an arm of the Institute of Medicine and the National Academy of Sciences. The National Academy of Sciences is a private, nonprofit society that was chartered by Congress in 1863 and serves to advise the federal government on scientific and technical topics.[40] The Institute of Medicine was established by the National Academy of Sciences in 1970 to examine matters related to the health of the public. Since 1941 the National Academy of Sciences has made periodic recommendations regarding the amounts of vitamins and minerals required to meet nutrient needs. This set of recommendations has historically been called the Recommended Dietary

Allowances, or RDAs. Including the latest version, eleven editions of these recommendations have been made.

Several changes in these recommendations have occurred throughout the years. However, the most significant change to date involves the 1997 version. First of all, the name has been changed from RDAs to Dietary Reference Intakes (DRIs). Secondly, in response to increasing evidence linking nutrition to conditions other than the classical nutrient deficiency diseases (such as scurvy and rickets), the National Academy of Sciences expanded its approach to nutrient intake recommendations by encompassing the potential role of nutrition in the prevention of chronic diseases. The 1997 recommendations also represent the first coordinated effort between the United States and Canada. In addition, the National Academy of Sciences recognizes that the recommended values can be used by individuals as a goal for intakes. The new calcium intake values from the National Academy of Sciences are as follows:

Ages 6 months or younger—210 mg

6 months to 1 year of age—270 mg

Ages 1 to 3 years—500 mg

Ages 4 to 8 years—800 mg

Ages 9 to 18 years—1,300 mg

Ages 19 to 50 years—1,000 mg

Ages 51 years or older—1,200 mg

CHAPTER TWO

Maximize Your Calcium Absorption

- Calcium and "Take-Home Pay"
- Food and Supplement Labels Don't Tell the Whole Story
- How the Body Absorbs Calcium
- The Importance of Calcium Solubility and Stomach Acidity
- Always Start and End the Day with Calcium
- Calcium Absorption from CCM
- Are Yogurt and Cheese As Good As Milk?
- Other Foods with Proven Calcium Absorption
- How to Get More from Your Calcium Supplement by Taking Less

Calcium absorption is an important feature to consider in deciding on the potential nutritional benefit of a calcium source. To be of value to your skeleton, the calcium you consume, whether it comes from foods, beverages, or supplements, must be absorbed. Not all calcium sources are created equal in terms of calcium absorption. In fact, there is quite a wide range of calcium absorption from one calcium source to another. In addition to selecting calcium sources with greater absorption, there are other ways you can improve your body's calcium absorption. These include taking calcium with meals, dividing your supplement dose into several smaller doses, and taking calcium at the right times during the day. In this chapter you'll learn how the body absorbs calcium, about the differences in calcium absorption from a wide variety of sources, and how to best use high-calcium foods and/or supplements to maximize their benefit.

Calcium and "Take-Home Pay"

Imagine having a job for which your take-home pay, due to taxes and other deductions from your paycheck, was only 25% of your gross salary. Not a very appealing situation, is it? Appealing or not, it accurately describes the situation that exists regarding calcium absorption by the human body. Think of the amount of calcium you consume from foods and supplements as your gross salary. However, the amount you absorb is what really counts; that's your calcium "take-home pay."

Unfortunately, most of the calcium you eat is not absorbed. In fact, a good working average for calcium absorption is about 25%. Simply put, this means your body only uses about 25% of the calcium you eat. The rest of the calcium, the other 75%, just passes through your gastrointestinal system and is eliminated. The good news is that not all calcium sources produce the same level of absorption. For example, although your body absorbs only 5% of the calcium contained in spinach, the calcium from CCM (whether you take it as a supplement or in a fortified beverage product) yields calcium absorption that is 40% greater than milk or calcium carbonate supplements (the most common type).[1–5]

Food and Supplement Labels Don't Tell the Whole Story

When you look at a label to find out how much calcium is in a food or calcium supplement, the value is typically presented as the % Daily Value, or %DV. Sometimes the manufacturers will also list the mg content of calcium. Currently, 100% of the daily value for calcium is equal to 1,000 mg. This value is set by the Food and Drug Administration (FDA). For example, if you look at the label on a bottle of milk, it will say calcium—30% Daily Value. This means that one serving of milk (8 ounces) contains 300 mg of calcium (30% of 1,000 mg).

There are at least two problems with letting the % Daily Value be your only guide for measuring the adequacy of calcium in your diet. First, it lists only one daily value for calcium; one size is supposed to fit all. Check the values at the end of Chapter 1, "How Much Calcium Do I Need?" You will see that different age groups have different recommended levels for calcium intake—or, in other words, one size does not fit all. For example, the calcium intake recommendation from the National Institutes of Health for a woman 50+ years of age is 1,500 mg—50% higher than the daily value used in food and supplement labeling.[6] So, even if you kept track of what you ate and the amount of calcium you consumed so that your total added up to 100% of the Daily Value, you would still be falling short of the recommended optimal intake. In fact, you would be getting only two-thirds of the calcium you need.

In addition to selecting calcium sources with greater absorption, there are other ways you can improve your body's calcium absorption. These include taking calcium with meals, dividing your supplement dose into several smaller doses, and taking calcium at the right times during the day.

The second problem with using the % Daily Value as your sole yardstick for measuring calcium intake is that it only describes the calcium content of the product. It doesn't take into account differences in calcium absorption. Remember, what really counts is the amount of *absorbed* calcium, not just the total calcium content. Using the example of milk again, an 8-ounce glass contains 300 mg of calcium. However, the absorption of calcium from a glass of milk is in the range of 25%–30%. Therefore, the amount of calcium that actually makes it into your system is about 75 mg.[2,7]

For milk, the most common food source of calcium in the American diet, the absorption rate is well-known. Calcium absorption from milk has been extensively studied and documented. Likewise, the most common source of supplemental calcium, calcium carbonate, has been thoroughly investigated and its calcium absorption is similar to milk.[2,7,8] Calcium carbonate is the source of the calcium found in the vast majority of supplements such as TUMS, Oscal, Caltrate, and many store brand supplements. However, manufacturers are not required to test calcium absorption. So for many food sources of calcium, we really don't know how well our bodies absorb the calcium in these products.

A number of natural food sources of calcium have been documented to have very good calcium absorption.[9] These include broccoli, kale, and brussels sprouts. However, the calcium content of these foods is relatively low compared to CCM-fortified beverages or dairy products. So even with the high absorption, they can't be relied on to shoulder most of your calcium needs. For example, to supply 500 mg of calcium, you need to eat 5 cups of cooked kale or 13 cups of brussels sprouts.

How the Body Absorbs Calcium

To reiterate, the calcium you consume must be *absorbed* in order to benefit your skeleton. To be absorbed, the calcium must be solubilized, or dissolved. The acid in your stomach, called hydrochloric acid, helps solubilize the calcium. However, no calcium is actually absorbed in the stomach but, rather, in the small intestine.

Unlike the stomach, the small intestine does not produce an acidic environment. Its lining is not designed to hold up to acid. For this reason, when the acidified contents of the stomach pass into the small intestine, they are rapidly neutralized by secretions that enter the small intestine. This means that calcium absorption takes place in the acid-neutral environment of the small intestine and that the solubility of calcium sources in an acid-neutral environment helps determine the level of absorption.

It's best to take your calcium supplement with a meal. Alternatively, you can use a soluble preparation of calcium, such as calcium citrate, or an even more soluble preparation such as CCM.

Different sources of calcium have widely different solubilities in an acid-neutral environment.[10] For example, CCM is 11 times more soluble than calcium citrate (used in some supplements and for food fortification), 82 times more soluble than tricalcium phosphate (also used in supplements and for food fortification), 571 times more soluble than calcium carbonate (the most common type of supplemental calcium and also used in food fortification), and 2,000 times more soluble than calcium oxalate (the type of calcium found in spinach).

Once calcium leaves the stomach, enters the small intestine, and is neutralized, it needs to be transported across the small intestine into the blood. This process is called calcium absorption. There are two possible pathways by which calcium is absorbed. Both involve moving calcium out of the small intestine and releasing it into the bloodstream. The first pathway is called *passive transport,* or *diffusion,* and involves the movement of the soluble calcium from an area of higher concentration (the intestine) to an area of lower concentration (the blood). You can think of this process as rolling a ball downhill—it requires no energy and occurs on its own without any special help. In this absorption pathway, calcium actually moves in-between the cells lining the intestine to find its way into the bloodstream.

The second pathway is called *active transport* and is like rolling a ball uphill. Active transport requires energy and a special helper protein called a *calcium-binding protein.* In this pathway, calcium moves into the lining of the intestinal cells and is shuttled across and into the blood by the helper protein. The intestinal cells' ability to manufacture calcium-binding protein is dependent on an activated form of vitamin D, called 1,25-dihydroxy vitamin D. It is different from the vitamin D found in supplements, milk, or other foods, or the vitamin D your body makes from exposure to sunlight (vitamin D is sometimes referred to as the "sunshine vitamin"). The vitamin D you eat or make from sunlight exposure is inactive to start with. Your body activates this vitamin D using specially designed enzymes in the liver and kidneys to make 1,25-dihydroxy vitamin D. That's why it's really a misnomer when people say that supplements with vitamin D are better absorbed. The vitamin D in all supplements is the inactive type and must be activated by your own body.

A special aspect of the active transport pathway for calcium absorption is it can react to changes in your dietary habits or your physiological state. During times when you need to be absorbing more calcium, your active transport pathway gears up to provide a greater degree of calcium absorption. For example, when you're pregnant or breastfeeding, active calcium transport increases. On the flip side, after women go through menopause, their reduced levels of estrogen make it more difficult for the body to activate vitamin D. As a result, their ability to absorb calcium goes down and their need for calcium intake goes up. That's one of the reasons why the calcium intake recommendation is increased dramatically for postmenopausal versus premenopausal women (1,500 versus 1,000 mg per day).

The Importance of Calcium Solubility and Stomach Acidity

Calcium in foods is present in various bound forms. To be absorbed, the food must be adequately digested in order to release the calcium and make it available. Similarly, calcium supplements made with insoluble forms of calcium, such as calcium carbonate (the most common type) and calcium phosphate, must be dissolved by acid in the stomach to liberate the calcium and make it available for absorption.

One of common challenges facing us as we age is a decrease in stomach acid production. As many as 30% to 40% of postmenopausal women have low to no stomach acid secretion unless the stomach is given some type of stimulus.[11] In addition, a considerable proportion of older individuals, both men and women, have lost the ability to produce stomach acid even when given a stimulus. The complete lack of ability to produce stomach acid is called achlorhydria. When people have a diminished ability to produce stomach acid but still produce a little, the condition is called hypochlorhydria.

Because calcium carbonate is the most frequently used source of supplemental calcium, and hypo- or achlorhydria is rather common, it's important to understand whether this insoluble calcium source can be used effectively under conditions of low stomach acid production.

A study published in the *New England Journal of Medicine* provides important insight to this issue.[11] The study consisted of 20 people with an average age of 60 years. Of the volunteers, 11 were verified to have achlorhydria and the other 9 had normal stomach acid production. Both groups received a 250-mg dose of calcium supplied as calcium carbonate or calcium citrate. Calcium citrate was chosen by the researchers because it is more soluble than calcium carbonate in a nonacid, or neutral, environment. This means that calcium citrate should be able to dissolve adequately even without the help of stomach acid. To be absolutely sure that the calcium citrate used in the study would be dissolved without the aid of stomach acid, the researchers predissolved it before the subjects took it.

To measure the degree of calcium absorption, the researchers used the "gold standard" method. This method is called the double-isotope, or dual-isotope, method because it involves giving two different types of radioactive calcium. Although there are several ways to measure calcium absorption, the double-isotope method is widely recognized as the most accurate. The amounts of the isotopes given are very small and safe. One isotope is mixed with the test dose and the other is given by intravenous injection. This method allows researchers to easily and accurately follow the calcium that's being tested. By comparing the amount of calcium isotope given intravenously (which represents 100% absorption because it all goes into the blood) to the amount that appears in the blood from the dose given orally (which needs to go from the gastrointestinal system into the blood by absorption), the amount of absorbed calcium can be calculated.

The results from this study clearly showed that calcium carbonate can be problematic for people with low stomach acid production. First, in the volunteers with normal stomach acid, there were no significant differences in calcium absorption between calcium carbonate and calcium citrate. This group also underwent a test in which milk was given as the source of calcium. *Again, there was no statistically significant difference in the absorption of calcium from milk, calcium carbonate, or calcium citrate. All three sources provided calcium that was absorbed between 22% and 26%.*

In the study volunteers with achlorhydria, calcium absorption from calcium carbonate was found to be very abnormal. *Only 5% of the calcium from calcium carbonate was absorbed.* To further investigate the lower calcium absorption from calcium carbonate, the researchers repeated the test but with one important change. Instead of giving the calcium carbonate on an empty stomach, they gave it along with a standard breakfast of eggs, toast, juice, and coffee. The effect of the meal was dramatic: Calcium absorption from calcium carbonate in the volunteers with achlorhydria increased to 21%.

Although the explanation of these findings is uncertain, it's clear that for older individuals or anyone who may have decreased stomach acid production, it's best to take your calcium supplement with a meal. Alternatively, you can use a soluble preparation of calcium, such as calcium citrate, or an even more soluble preparation such as CCM (11 times more soluble than calcium citrate). Also, CCM, taken as a supplement or in beverages, is a good choice because it is clinically proven to yield greater absorption than calcium carbonate, even when calcium carbonate is taken with a meal.[5,6,8]

Always Start and End the Day with Calcium

In addition to being the basic building block of your skeleton, calcium is absolutely vital to many other processes in your body. About 99% of your body's calcium is located in the bones and teeth. The other 1% is in the blood, in the membranes of cells, inside all the cells, and in the fluid bathing the cells.

Calcium is needed for muscle contraction, nerve conduction, blood clotting, regulating how permeable your cell membranes are, helping to signal the internal workings of your cells to what's happening outside, and a whole host of other functions. Because of the vital role that calcium plays during virtually every second of your existence, the concentration of calcium in the blood is very tightly regulated by various hormones. Too little or too much calcium in the blood can be lethal. If your intake of calcium from either diet or supplements is insufficient to maintain normal blood calcium concentrations, your body responds by tapping into its own calcium bank—your bones. An important hormone involved in the regulation of blood calcium and the removal of calcium from the skeleton is called parathyroid hormone, or PTH for short.

As the name implies, PTH is made in the parathyroid gland. The relationship between PTH and the control of blood calcium concentration was first noted in 1925. Since that time, a great deal has been learned about the actions of this hormone. It has been clearly established that the main factor causing the secretion of PTH is low calcium concentration in our extracellular fluids (the blood and other fluids that bathe our cells). PTH has a triple-action mechanism for increasing the calcium concentration in blood. First, PTH stimulates the release of calcium from the bones into the blood. Second, PTH causes our kidneys to pass less calcium into the urine as they filter our blood. Third, PTH stimulates the enzyme needed to make active vitamin D, which, in turn, helps boost our absorption of calcium in the small intestine.

Without a steady supply of calcium from what we eat, blood calcium concentration will begin to drop. This causes an increase in PTH and the removal of calcium from the skeleton. That's why it's important not to skip meals during the day and to be sure all your meals contain adequate amounts of calcium. Sometimes it may just be impossible for you to eat at regular intervals or to have adequate control over the foods that are available. For these circumstances, I recommend that you carry a small supply of calcium supplements with you at all times to take care of these emergency needs.

Even if you can always control when and what you can eat, there is a time each day when you go without a supply of calcium. When you sleep at night, you are fasting. Your body has no readily available supply of calcium except for the calcium in your bones. Not surprisingly, there is a well-documented nighttime rise in PTH as the body struggles to keep its blood calcium level at normal concentrations. PTH concentrations are greatest in the morning, right after you get up, because your body has been tapping into your skeletal calcium supply while you sleep. To help control the harmful effect to your bones from the nighttime rise in PTH, do two things: First, consume a high calcium-containing food or take one of your daily calcium supplement doses before bedtime. This will give you a supply of calcium while you sleep and should help blunt the nighttime rise in PTH. Second, be sure your breakfast contains a high calcium food or calcium supplement. After your overnight fast, you need to get some calcium into your system to prevent taking calcium from your bones. This approach, calcium at bedtime and first thing in the morning, has a double benefit. Not only will it help reduce the increase in PTH and the leaching of calcium from your bones, but it will also ensure that you divide your total calcium intake into at least two doses during the day. Taking calcium in several smaller doses throughout the day results in much more absorbed calcium than one large dose taken all at once.

Calcium Absorption from CCM

During the mid-1980s, the time when the first calcium absorption research began on CCM, the thinking in the scientific and medical communities was that all calcium sources produced the same level of absorption. There were two important studies conducted during that time that helped foster this belief. The first study compared calcium absorption from milk, other dairy products, and calcium carbonate in a group of 10 women between the ages of 40 and 70. The report, which was published in the *American Journal of Clinical Nutrition,* showed no significant differences among the calcium sources.[7] The average calcium absorption from all the test products was 24%. The second study, published in the *New England Journal of Medicine,* compared the absorption of calcium from several supplemental sources of calcium in a group of eight healthy young men.[8] The sources tested included calcium carbonate, calcium citrate, calcium lactate, calcium gluconate, and calcium acetate. Milk was also evaluated as a control sample. Again, no difference was found in calcium absorption among these test products. None of them were significantly better or worse than milk.

Taking calcium in several smaller doses throughout the day results in much more absorbed calcium than one large dose taken all at once.

Given the results from these two important studies, we predicted that calcium absorption from CCM would be equivalent to milk and calcium carbonate. A research study was designed to make these comparisons in healthy young women, ages 21 to 30. The study was conducted at Creighton University in Omaha, Nebraska. The first part of the study compared calcium absorption from supplement tablets made from CCM or calcium carbonate in groups of 10 women each. The second half of the study compared absorption of calcium from milk to absorption from a beverage (orange juice) fortified with CCM, in groups of 12 women each.

To our great surprise, the results of this study showed highly significant differences in favor of CCM. *The degree of cal-*

cium absorption from CCM was 26% greater than that of calcium carbonate and 30% greater than that of milk. We had apparently found an exception to the rule that all calcium sources were created equal. The results of this study were published in a journal called *Calcified Tissue International* and led to additional research on calcium absorption from CCM.[2] A follow-up study was conducted at the Indiana University School of Medicine in Indianapolis and focused on calcium absorption from CCM in groups of older women (average age—57 years). It was important to test whether the same high level of calcium absorption from CCM was observed in older women because the ability to absorb calcium is known to decrease with age. Both orange juice and apple juice were fortified with CCM in amounts that equaled the same level of calcium found in milk. A total of 114 women participated in the study. Once again, the results showed excellent performance from CCM.[1] The average calcium absorption equaled 39.0%, *a value that is 30%–50% greater than is typically found for milk.* These results were published in the *Journal of the American College of Nutrition.*

As it is with adults, a key to optimizing bone health during childhood is to consume highly absorbable sources of calcium on a daily basis. Following the results we obtained with CCM in adults, we wondered whether the same advantage could be found in children. If so, then another tool would be available to help ensure better bone health during the important years of growth and development. Highly absorbable, clinically proven calcium sources are certainly needed during this time of life. About 50% of our total adult bone mass is built during puberty. However, calcium intake typically falls off during the teenage years as kids' food preferences begin to change and parents are less able to exercise control over what they eat. Nationwide, about 75% of boys and 90%–95%

of teenage girls consume less than the recommended amount of calcium.[12]

Nationwide, about 75% of boys and 90%–95% of teenage girls consume less than the recommended amount of calcium.

To see whether CCM would give adolescent children an advantage in calcium absorption, a group of 12 healthy children (6 boys and 6 girls), average age 14 years, participated in a study comparing CCM to calcium carbonate.[3] The kids served as their own controls in the study by taking both supplements at different times. As was seen for adults, the results with CCM were very significant. On average, calcium absorption was 37% greater from CCM than from calcium carbonate. This study was a joint research effort conducted with the Indiana University School of Medicine and Purdue University. It was published in the *American Journal of Clinical Nutrition* in 1988. A year later, another study conducted in conjunction with the same two universities was published, comparing calcium absorption from CCM and calcium carbonate in children.[4] The results were confirmed and even larger differences were seen! *This time, calcium absorption from CCM exceeded calcium carbonate by 55%.*

Overall, the research conducted on calcium absorption from CCM has clearly established it as one of the most bioavailable (absorbable) calcium sources currently accessible to children or adults. Taking into account all the studies done with CCM as both a calcium supplement and in the form of CCM-fortified beverages, CCM's advantage over calcium carbonate and milk averages about 40% more absorbed calcium on a mg-for-mg basis. As you will learn in later chapters of this book, this absorption advantage for CCM can translate into very meaningful long-term benefits for bone health throughout the life cycle.

Are Yogurt and Cheese As Good As Milk?

Currently, dairy products are the main source of calcium in the American diet. Within the dairy group, fluid milk is by far the most common source of calcium. National statistics show that the younger you are, the more milk you drink. For example, grade-school age girls drink a little over one cup per day. By the time they reach the teenage years, this has dropped to less than a cup. This trend continues so that, on average, the typical American woman consumes about 4.5 ounces of milk per day and the typical man about 6 ounces.[13] One of the great misconceptions that people have concerning the adequacy of their calcium intake is that if they drink milk, they're meeting their calcium nutritional needs. However, current volumes of milk consumption only supply about one-sixth the recommended amount of calcium for women and one-fifth the recommended amount for men. Milk on your cereal in the morning, or in your coffee, or even a full glass of milk just doesn't go very far toward supplying the total recommended amount. A serving of milk is a nice foundation to build on. However, since most of us aren't willing or able to boost our milk intake up to several servings a day, we need to get smarter about the other good sources of calcium available from the dairy group as well as from calcium-fortified foods and supplements.

With the additional variety of products being added to the yogurt and cheese cases in the grocery store, it's important to understand how these dairy products differ from milk. The two main factors to consider are their calcium absorption and calcium content. For calcium absorption, the situation is pretty easy. A study was conducted several years ago to measure the calcium absorption from different dairy products.[7] As an added bonus, a calcium carbonate supplement was also included. The following calcium absorption values were obtained:

Milk—26.7%

Yogurt—25.4%

Chocolate milk—23.2%

Cheese—22.9%

Calcium carbonate—22.0%

Although the values for these products fall well below what has been found for CCM products (36%–42% calcium absorption), at least you know that when it comes to different dairy sources, they all perform about the same for calcium absorption. Thus, you can use them interchangeably, from a calcium absorption standpoint, to help meet your daily calcium needs.

The second factor to consider is the calcium content of different dairy products. There are a lot of misconceptions on this topic, so let's get to the facts.[14] First of all, there is very little difference in the calcium content of whole milk, 2% milk, skim milk, and, for that matter, chocolate milk or even buttermilk. They all contain about 280 to 300 mg of calcium per 8 fluid ounces (one cup). There is, however, a big difference between them in their calorie count. Skim milk comes in at about 86 calories per cup, 2% has 121 calories, whole milk (3.3% fat) has 150 calories, and chocolate milk, even if it's made with 2% milk, has 179 calories. The extra calories in the chocolate variety come from added sugar.

Yogurt can vary tremendously in calcium content, depending on the type and brand you purchase. That's because the package sizes are not all the same and the amounts of non-yogurt ingredients (fruit fillings, flavorings, etc.) are not all the same. In other words, the amount of yogurt you actually get in a single-serving-size container is different. My own personal favorite is plain nonfat yogurt, the most concentrated source of yogurt calcium. One cup gives you 400 mg of calcium and only contains 120 calories. Generally speaking, the fruit-flavored types of yogurt contain somewhere between 200 and 350 mg of calcium. Be sure to check the labels so you can accurately compare calcium content.

Cheese varies even more in calcium content than do yogurt products. In general, the harder the cheese is, the more calcium it has. At opposite ends of the spectrum are cream cheese, a very soft cheese with 23 mg of calcium per ounce, and parmesan cheese, a very hard cheese with 340 mg of calcium per ounce. Some of the other more popular cheeses include Swiss (272 mg/ounce), Cheddar (204 mg/ounce), and American (174 mg/ounce). Cottage cheese (2% milk fat) has about 150 mg of calcium per one-cup serving. If you're concerned with fat and calories, look for the reduced-fat versions of cheeses.

Frozen desserts, like ice cream and frozen yogurt, are fun to eat and reasonably rich sources of calcium as well. Remember, milk is a main starting ingredient for many of these items. Plain old regular vanilla ice cream contains 176 mg of calcium per cup. Soft-serve vanilla has 377 mg of calcium per cup and orange sherbet comes in at 103 mg of calcium per cup. Of course, if you're watching your fat and calorie intake, you'd be wise to reach for the low-fat varieties, which have as much, if not more, calcium. Also, be on the lookout for calcium-fortified dairy products; yogurt, milk, cottage cheese, and even frozen yogurt varieties are available in most grocery stores. These products are typically fortified with calcium carbonate, calcium phosphate, or calcium lactate. Although there is no special value to the sources of calcium used to fortify these products, they do, at least, have boosted levels of calcium.

Other Foods with Proven Calcium Absorption

Once you get past dairy products and fortified foods, there aren't many other food products that supply high levels of calcium. Within the dairy group, we know that milk, yogurt, and many cheeses are concentrated sources of calcium and that the calcium in them is absorbed at a moderate level. With respect to fortified foods, little is known about the calcium absorption from these products. The exceptions are products fortified with CCM, which we know display high levels of calcium absorption.

Fruits are generally very low in calcium and little is known about the absorption of calcium from them. The same goes for meat products, which contain very little calcium. One exception to this is canned fish with bones, such as sardines. That's because you get the calcium from the bones, not the flesh. A 3-ounce serving of sardines contains 370 mg of calcium (if you eat the bones). Although the calcium absorption from sardine bones has not been measured, calcium absorption from cow bones and from calcium phosphate supplements, which resemble bones in their composition, have been assessed. Calcium absorption from these products is from 10% to 80% less absorbable than absorption from calcium carbonate and milk.[10]

The other foods that can contribute to your total calcium intake are vegetables. As you will see, some of these vegetables possess very high estimates for calcium absorption. However, even the richest ones are fairly low in calcium content compared to dairy and CCM-fortified products. That means you need to eat a large quantity to get the total absorbable calcium you require. Nevertheless, vegetables are clearly an important part of any healthy, well-balanced diet. In fact, the National Cancer Institute recognizes that increasing the amount of fruits and vegetables you consume may lower your risk of cancer. They specifically single out vegetables from the cabbage family (cruciferous vegetables) as being of particular importance. Fortunately, this same group of vegetables tends to be one of the highest in terms of calcium content and absorption.

Although a complete survey of calcium absorption from vegetable products has yet to be done, a fairly wide range of vegetables, including legumes and nuts, have been assessed for calcium absorption by researchers at Purdue University.[9] Their information was published in a very convenient way, listing the factors of both calcium content and calcium absorption. By combining the calcium content of the foods with their estimates

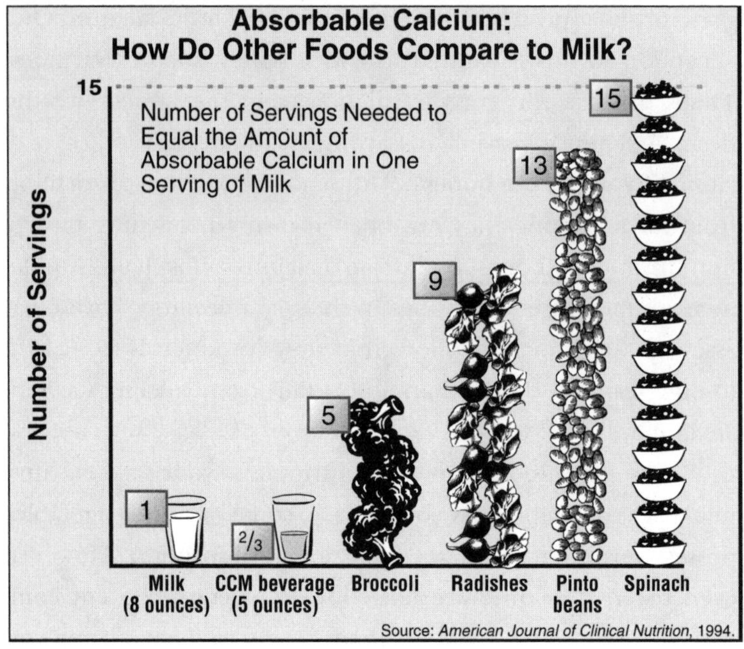

Figure 2-1

You only need ⅔ of a serving of a CCM beverage to get the same amount of absorbable calcium in a full serving of milk.

for calcium absorption, they calculated the amount of absorbed calcium that will be derived from a serving of the individual foods. Furthermore, by comparing these results to what is known about milk calcium absorption, they calculated the number of servings of a food that you must consume to equal the amount of absorbed calcium from one 8-ounce glass of milk. The results of this work first appeared in the *American Journal of Clinical Nutrition* and included information on CCM-fortified beverages and several other foods (see Figure 2-1). As you read about their discoveries, keep in mind that a standard serving of vegetables equals one-half cup.

Spinach: Spinach has long been touted by some nutritionists as a good alternative source of calcium. As vegetables go, it is one of the highest in calcium content. However, calcium absorption tests show that it is one of worst, if not *the* worst, foods to turn to for supplying calcium. Despite the fact that a definitive study on this topic has been completed, I still see newspaper and magazine articles suggesting that people eat spinach as a good source of calcium. Researchers compared spinach and milk and found that the corresponding calcium absorptions from these products were 5.1% and 27.6%, respectively. In addition, although a serving of spinach has more calcium than many vegetables, it has much less than a serving of milk. The net result is that you need to eat 15 to 16 servings of spinach to equal the amount of absorbed calcium from one glass of milk.

Nuts and Seeds: Dry roasted almonds and sesame seeds have been evaluated for calcium absorption and are nearly identical. Percentage of calcium absorption was estimated at 21.2% for almonds and 20.8% for sesame seeds. However, on an ounce-for-ounce basis, almonds have about twice as much calcium. Compared to one glass of milk, you need to eat 6 one-ounce servings of almonds and 12 one-ounce servings of sesame seeds to yield the same amount of absorbable calcium.

Beans: Calcium absorption from three varieties of beans (pinto beans, red beans, and white beans) was estimated to be 17.0%. Taking into account the different calcium contents of the bean varieties, the number of servings of beans needed to equal the amount of absorbed calcium from a glass of milk are 12.7 servings of pinto beans, 14 servings of red beans, or 5 servings of white beans.

Radishes, Rutabagas, and Kohlrabi: Although your chance of regularly eating these vegetables is quite low, their calcium absorption numbers are quite high. Calcium absorption for radishes was estimated at 74.4%, rutabagas at 61.4%, and kohlrabi at 67.0%. The amounts you need to eat to equal the absorbed calcium from a glass of milk are 4.5 cups of radishes, 2.5 cups of rutabagas, and 3.5 cups of kohlrabi.

Cabbage Family (Cruciferous Vegetables): Calcium absorption from regular cabbage (green cabbage) and Chinese cabbage (bok choy) were found to be high, 64.9% and 53.8%, respectively. However, the Chinese variety contains slightly more than three times as much calcium per serving. To equal the absorbed calcium from milk, you need to eat about 2.5 servings of bok choy or 6 servings of cabbage. Other cruciferous vegetables with high calcium absorption estimates were found to be broccoli (52.6%), brussels sprouts (63.8%), cauliflower (68.6%), and kale (58.8%). To get the same amount of absorbed calcium from one serving of milk, eat the following quantities of the these vegetables—5 servings of broccoli, 8 servings of brussels sprouts, 8 servings of cauliflower, or 3.5 servings of kale.

Soy Milk and Tofu: Soybean-based products are an integral part of some Asian diets and are beginning to grow in popularity in the United States. According to information published in the *Journal of Nutrition,* there are at least two emerging areas of research for the potential health benefits of soy products that warrant further study. First, soy has been shown to have cholesterol-lowering effects. Second, there is clearly evidence to suggest that soy may be protective against several types of cancer, including breast cancer. Estimates for calcium absorption from soy milk (unfortified) and tofu (calcium-set) were 5.1% and 31.0%, respectively. Soy itself is quite low in calcium. Thus, to get any real calcium benefit, you need to eat calcium-set tofu, in which calcium sulfate is added to help coagulate the soy proteins. One to 1.5 servings of calcium-set tofu will yield the absorbable calcium of a glass of milk. Soy milk requires a whopping 60 servings because of its poor absorption and very low calcium content. Calcium-fortified soy milks are available but have not been evaluated with respect to their calcium absorption.

CCM-Fortified Beverages: CCM-fortified beverages were also included in this survey and produced some very exciting results. As you no doubt noticed in reviewing the results of these absorption studies, even the best-absorbed calcium sources from vegetables require several servings at once to equal the absorbed calcium from a glass of milk. That's because their calcium content is relatively low compared to milk. The exceptions to this are CCM-fortified beverages, which have as much calcium, ounce for ounce, as milk. In addition, the estimated calcium absorption from CCM products in the food product survey was greater compared to milk (51.0% versus 32.1%). Thus, the estimated number of servings of a CCM-fortified beverage you need to consume to equal the absorbable calcium in a glass of milk is less than one. According to the published results from the survey, 5.3 ounces of a CCM-fortified beverage will deliver the same amount of absorbable calcium as an 8-ounce glass of milk.

Maximize Your Calcium Absorption

How to Get More from Your Calcium Supplement by Taking Less

Whether it's calcium from a food or a supplement, we all want to get the most calcium we can out of it. What most people don't realize is that more calcium is not always better when it comes to maximizing absorption. As a matter of convenience, many women take their supplemental calcium all at once. Furthermore, they may be taking their supplements in the morning along with a breakfast that consists of cereal with milk. The end result of this pattern of intake is they consume most of their total calcium for the day at one time. Although this practice is certainly better than doing nothing at all, it will place you at a disadvantage for getting the most benefit out of the calcium you consume.

The smaller the amount of calcium you eat at one time, the greater your absorption will be. The absorption pathways your body uses for calcium have their limits in terms of how much calcium they can handle at one time. Put another way, it's fairly easy to saturate your body's ability to absorb calcium from a single meal or single dose of supplemental calcium. As you approach this level of saturation, you hit a point of diminishing returns for calcium absorption and start to waste calcium. Remember, humans have a fairly low ability for absorbing calcium to begin with. In general, our absorption efficiency—the percentage of calcium we actually absorb out of the total amount we consume—is only about 25%. Thus, it's important to use your supplement or high-calcium-containing food selections in a way that maximizes your chance of absorbing calcium.

The basic relationship between the amount of calcium consumed at one time and the percentage of that calcium that is absorbed was noted during early studies of calcium absorption. However, a systematic study of this relationship was not conducted until 1990 (the study is described in the following paragraphs). As you will see, this relationship has a dramatic impact on the amount of calcium you utilize. This is particularly true when it comes to maximizing absorption from calcium supplements because they are often formulated to contain 500 mg or more of calcium. In comparison, the very richest sources of calcium in foods or beverages typically do not contain more than about 300 mg of calcium per serving.

Twenty-four healthy adult women volunteered to help investigate the effect of different doses of calcium on the percentage of absorption.[15] They consumed the calcium test doses along with a light meal, which tends to improve absorption and eliminate the possible negative effect of low stomach acid production. Although milk was used as the source of calcium for the study, the results apply to other common sources of calcium from food or supplements.

The results of the study showed a strong relationship between the amount of calcium consumed and the percentage of the calcium absorbed. To illustrate this point, let's use calcium carbonate as an example. Calcium carbonate is the most common type of calcium used in supplements. A good average value for its percentage of calcium absorption at a 250-mg dose is 26%. That means that of the 250 mg of calcium you take in the calcium carbonate supplement, you absorb only 65 mg (26% of 250 mg = 65 mg). Now, using the relationship between dose and percentage of calcium absorption found in the study, it can be calculated that if you took 1,000 mg of calcium as calcium carbonate, your percentage of absorption would be only 14.9% (remember, as the dose goes up, the percentage of absorption goes down). So, the amount of calcium you actually absorb from the 1,000-mg dose equals 149 mg (14.9% of 1,000 mg = 149 mg).

Now let's compare two different ways of taking 1,000 mg of supplemental calcium as calcium carbonate. As I showed earlier, if you take the 1,000 mg of calcium all at once, you only get 149 mg of absorbed calcium. However, if you take a 250-mg dose at four different times during the day, your total absorbed calcium will be 260 mg (four times 65 mg). Actually, you'd get more absorbed calcium by taking 750 mg of calcium spread out as three 250-doses than you would from a single 1,000-mg dose.

The same principles of absorption apply to food sources of calcium. If you choose to exclusively use foods to meet your daily demands for calcium, you should consume a rich source with every meal. In this way your total calcium intake is spread out during the day and absorption will be greater. Of course, using CCM, with its greater absorption factor, will give you an advantage at any dose schedule you choose. For example, consuming four separate 250-mg doses of calcium as CCM, with a 40% absorption factor, produces 400 mg of absorbed calcium. The CCM approach for getting more absorbable calcium has another advantage as well. As you will read in Chapter 6 on the dangers of too much calcium, common sources of calcium (foods and supplements) have been shown to reduce the absorption of other minerals such as iron, zinc, and magnesium. Thus, if you ramp up your dosage amounts to compensate for the lower bioavailability of some calcium sources, you increase the chance of blocking these other minerals.

CHAPTER THREE

Osteoporosis—Too Little of a Good Thing

- **Defining the Problem**
- **Fractures—When and Where Are They Going to Happen?**
- **More Than Just a Physical Problem**
- **Importance of Family History and Genetics**
- **Lifestyle Factors That Impact Risk**
- **Estrogen Therapy**

Osteoporosis literally means "porous bone." It is characterized by having too little bone, although whatever bone tissue you do have is normal (i.e., too little of a good thing). Osteoporosis currently affects at least 25 million Americans. It contributes to 1.5 million fractures per year and costs our medical care system an estimated $10–$20 billion per year.[1,2] A woman's lifetime risk of developing a hip fracture is slightly higher than her combined risk of developing breast, uterine, and ovarian cancers.[2,3] For a man, the lifetime risk of hip fracture is the same as his chances of developing prostate cancer.[3] Mortality after a hip fracture has been reported to be as high as 30% during the first year after the fracture, and in the majority of these cases, death comes within three months following the fracture.[1] About 50% of those who survive a hip fracture and go through rehabilitation will shift from an independent to dependent lifestyle.[3] This chapter will help define when osteoporosis is present, the physical and emotional complications to expect if you become osteoporotic, and the most important risk factors for osteoporosis prevention.

Defining the Problem

Osteoporosis is the most common bone disease in the world. In the past, some referred to it as "brittle bone disease," although it is now more accurately referred to as "fragile bone disease." Increased longevity, more emphasis on women's health issues, the aging of the baby boom generation, and technology advancements in accurately and painlessly measuring bone density have helped bring this once-anonymous disease to the forefront.

Osteoporosis is also known as "the silent thief" because the body robs itself of bone tissue during an insidious process without overt symptoms. This bone-robbing process proceeds slowly, but continuously, over many years in both men and women. The most visible tell-tale sign of osteoporosis in our society is the loss of height that occurs with aging. We all know that as people get older, they seem to shrink. It's not uncommon to be taken aback by the small stature of an older parent or relative you haven't visited for a while. In return, that older relative sees it from a different perspective and may ask whether somehow you are growing taller. Some of this apparent loss in height is due to the poor postural changes that occur with aging; however, much of it is from a partial compression of the vertebral bodies in the spine and is characteristic of osteoporosis. We don't shrink because our legs are getting shorter but because our spinal column is compressing due to lack of bone strength in the vertebrae.

Osteoporosis is also known as "the silent thief" because the body robs itself of bone tissue during an insidious process without overt symptoms. This bone-robbing process proceeds slowly, but continuously, over many years in both men and women.

Although we have some evidence that osteoporosis existed in centuries past, its prevalence was not known until recently. Like many of the chronic diseases that currently plague our society, osteoporosis appears to be a by-product of the lifestyle changes brought about through technological and cultural advances. Most notably, our increasing life span has provided the necessary backdrop for osteoporosis to become an all-too-common condition. Our bones generally reach their peak density and strength before the age of 30 and begin to decline thereafter. At some skeletal sites, such as the hip and spine, the peak may be reached as early as age 20.[4] In earlier, less "civilized" times, we were unlikely to live long enough to develop osteoporosis. Death from infection, childbirth, traumatic injury, and a host of other conditions that are now treatable (or, at least, manageable) were much more common.

Our bones generally reach their peak density and strength before the age of 30 and begin to decline thereafter. At some skeletal sites, such as the hip and spine, the peak may be reached as early as age 20.

There are several clinical definitions for osteoporosis. Most of these involve some measure of bone density and the concept of a fracture threshold, or the amount of bone below which our risk for fracture increases. Although much has been written about the fracture threshold, and it is a convenient way to mentally picture and clinically classify osteoporosis risk, it may not adequately define the problem of osteoporosis. According to Christopher Nordin, M.D., University of Adelaide, Australia (one of the world's foremost leaders in the area of osteoporosis and calcium metabolism), the risk for osteoporotic fracture is an unbroken continuum related to bone density.[5] In other words, your bones can fracture with a bone density above the so-called fracture threshold, and conversely, you can be fracture-free below the threshold. The important thing is to limit your risk for fracture, which, for every individual at every age, will always be lower if bone density is higher.

A big problem with cultivating an awareness of osteoporosis and managing your risk is that many people believe, and some medical definitions include, the presence of a fracture as a prerequisite for the diagnosis of osteoporosis. Given the insidious, slowly progressing nature of bone loss, this attitude is tremendously counterproductive for getting people to understand the disease and take steps to manage it. To wait until fractures begin before diagnosing osteoporosis would be like waiting for a heart attack to occur before diagnosing elevated cholesterol levels. The simple fact is that once our peak bone density is reached and bone loss begins in adulthood, all of us start down that slippery slope toward osteoporosis with increased risk of fracture. If you can build more bone density when you're young, then you have a longer distance to slide and a better chance of keeping risk low. Also, if you can change the angle of the slope, or flatten it out, then you can reduce or slow the bone loss process and thereby keep risk to a minimum.

Fractures—When and Where Are They Going to Happen?

Osteoporotic fractures are becoming more and more common as the number of older people in our population continues to increase. All parts of the skeleton are susceptible to osteoporosis, except, perhaps, the skull, which tends to increase in density with age. However, the most common fractures in older persons occur at the wrist, spine, and hip (see Figure 3-1). The number of wrist fractures in women starts to go up at the time of menopause. The increase in the fracture rate is very sharp so that women in their 60s have an incidence of wrist fractures 7 to 20 times higher than that of women in their 30s.[1,6]

The incidence of vertebral fractures is difficult to measure because people don't always know when they get them. Pain in the back, per se, is not evidence of a vertebral fracture and, conversely, a vertebral fracture does not always cause pain. Other conditions can cause a similar type of pain, such as muscle strain, disc problems, and arthritis. In fact, many vertebral fractures cause no, or very little, pain. It's been estimated that as many as two-thirds of all vertebral fractures are not brought to the attention of a doctor.[1] This is part of the insidious nature of osteoporosis. Bone loss itself occurs with no overt symptoms, and even vertebral fractures, the most common type of osteoporotic fracture, can occur without any sign or warning. The first whiff of trouble can be when a woman begins to notice a loss of height or the development of a curved back. Of course, by this time, a substantial amount of bone density has been lost over a long period of time.

Vertebral fractures are different from the fracture of a long bone in the arm or leg. Vertebral fractures are often referred to as collapsed, or compression, fractures. Different parts of the same vertebrae may suddenly compress at different times during a period lasting months or years. Thus, the same vertebrae may experience many separate fracture episodes, with the end result being a partially or fully collapsed shape. Vertebral compression fractures are the most common osteo-

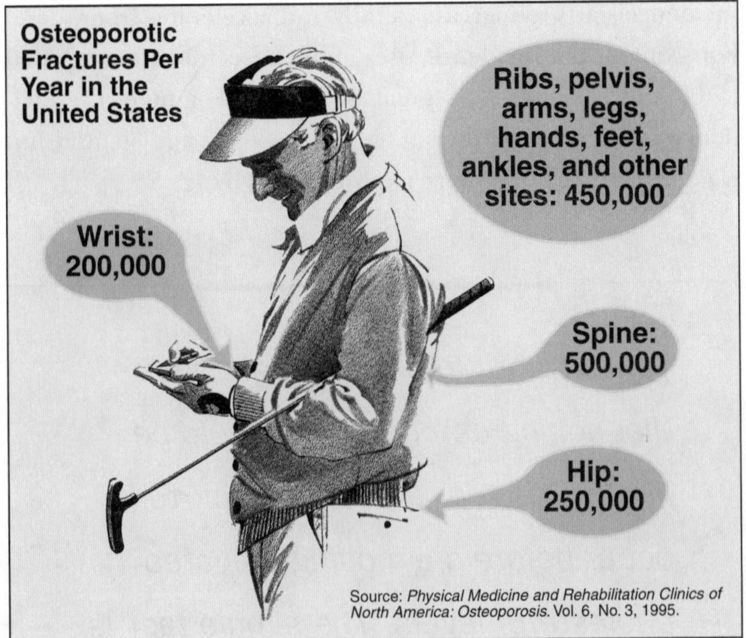

Source: *Physical Medicine and Rehabilitation Clinics of North America: Osteoporosis.* Vol. 6, No. 3, 1995.

Figure 3-1

porosis-related fractures in women and occur mainly after menopause. The incidence of vertebral compression fractures increases approximately eightfold from the ages of 50 to 85. Sixty percent of women over the age of 70 have at least one compression fracture.[1]

Hip fractures are the most disastrous type of osteoporotic fracture, accounting for most of the medical costs of the disease. Mortality (death) after a hip fracture has been reported to be as high as 30% during the first year following the fracture. The incidence of hip fracture begins to rise after about 50 years of age in both men and women; however, the rate of increase is very slow at first. At about 60 to 65 years of age, the incidence starts to increase rapidly and accelerates from there. For women, the incidence rises about threefold from ages 50 to 60 and is 15 times as great by age 75. For men, the incidence is 2.5 times greater at age 60 versus at age 50, and hip fractures are 22 times more likely to occur by age 75.[1,6]

To wait until fractures begin before diagnosing osteoporosis would be like waiting for a heart attack to occur before diagnosing elevated cholesterol levels. The simple fact is that once our peak bone density is reached and bone loss begins in adulthood, all of us start down that slippery slope toward osteoporosis with increased risk of fracture.

What About Men?

Osteoporosis is the only chronic disease for which research in men has been underrepresented. It is clearly an important, but currently under-appreciated, public health problem for men. The risk of fractures in men is lower than in women. Depending on the skeletal site, men are about two to five times less likely to suffer an osteoporotic fracture. Men have about 30% more peak skeletal mass and don't go through a rapid bone loss phase immediately after menopause as women do. Thus, men have a built-in protective advantage against osteoporosis. Men have another "advantage" over women when it comes to osteoporosis—they die sooner. This means they are less likely to reach a point of bone fragility when the risk of fracture substantially increases. However, when men's bones do fracture, it's often more serious because men are in poorer general health than women at the time of the fracture. For example, the risk of hip fracture in older men is about one-half that of older women. However, their risk of death following the fracture is about twice as high.[7]

More Than Just a Physical Problem

An often overlooked and greatly underestimated aspect of osteoporosis is its effect on an individual's quality of life. I've been describing osteoporosis from a more global perspective up until this point, in terms of the incidence of different fractures in the population and the cost of this disease to our medical care system. However, besides the obvious physical disabilities that accompany osteoporosis, there are important psychological and social changes that occur to further diminish one's quality of life.[8] These factors involve the emotional aspects of the disease and its practical ramifications in everyday life. They are, in a sense, much more important than the sterile statistics concerning risk of fracture, fracture rates, and medical costs.

The risk of hip fracture in older men is about one-half that of older women. However, their risk of death following the fracture is about twice as high.

How, and to what extent, osteoporosis will affect your quality of life depends on your individual circumstances. The black-and-white clinical studies defining the severity of osteoporosis do not go hand in hand with a decrease of functioning in everyday life. A study of vertebral osteoporosis conducted by researchers in the Department of Medicine at McMaster University in Ontario, Canada, found there was little, if any, relationship between a woman's number of fractures and the extent of her pain, negative emotions, and loss of participation in the activities of daily living.[9] Thus, the degree to which an individual suffers in terms of quality of life factors is not directly related to the severity of the disease.

Like any other chronic condition that adversely affects health, osteoporosis requires individuals to make certain adjustments in their daily routines. These changes impact the way they interact with people and how they view themselves and their place in society and in their families. For example, women have traditionally been the caregivers in a family. They function as doctor, counselor, chief cook, and bottlewasher, all rolled into one. However, the physical conditions and associated limitations that come with osteoporosis, such as chronic pain, limited range of motion, and muscle fatigue, may cause them to shift from the care-giving role within the family to a more helpless state in which *they* must be taken care of. Along with this shift in responsibility comes a shift in attitude and self-perception. Feelings of dependency, of being a burden to others, frustration, and even anger are common.

By surveying a group of women who reported persistent pain due to vertebral fractures from osteoporosis, the researchers at McMaster University were able to quantitate and classify the common quality of life issues these women faced.[9] A profile emerged of a woman living not only in pain, but also in anger, frustration, and fear. She's not able to do normal everyday activities as well as she once could and needs the help of others to just get by. Many women (70%–87%) reported difficulty in bending over, walking, lifting, and carrying things. Shopping for food and clothing was affected in 60% of the women studied; vacuuming and doing housework was affected in 81% and 70%, respectively. Emotionally, 82% of the women had a fear of falling or of incurring a fracture (74%). Negative feelings are common in women with spinal osteoporosis—feelings such as frustration (66%), anger (53%), and being overwhelmed (49%). Activities that should bring joy into their lives are limited. About 33% of the women had difficulty going to church, 57% had trouble traveling, and something as simple as finding a comfortable chair was affected in 68% of the women. All of these factors combined lead to a lifestyle of less social interaction and less physical activity. This, in turn, contributes to

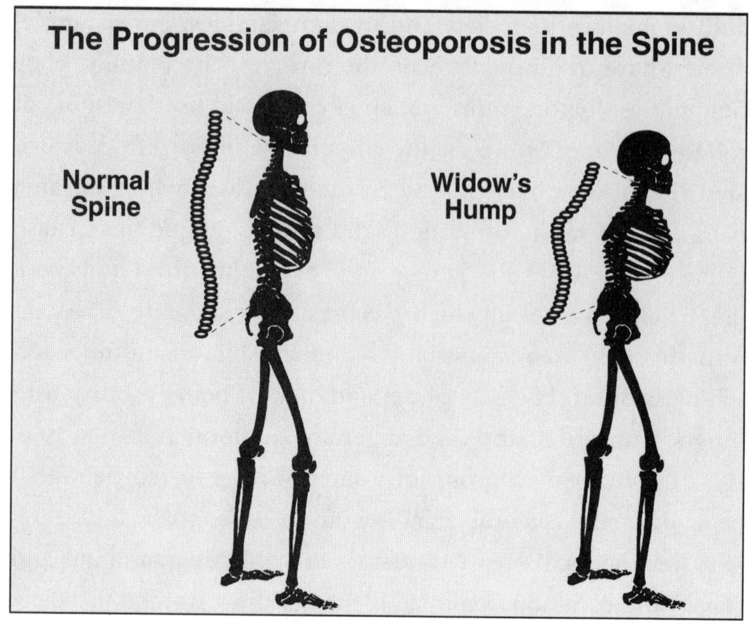

Figure 3-2

further bone loss and muscle weakness caused by disuse, which increases the risk for additional fractures and falls.

Vertebral fractures cause a change in appearance in addition to the loss of height. The marked rounding of the upper back and shoulder area, which is common as osteoporosis progresses, is a type of physical deformity that can cause embarrassment. "Dorsal kyphosis" is the medical term for what is more commonly called the "dowager's hump" or "widow's hump" (see Figure 3-2). This stooped posture and humped back is caused because vertebrae tend to collapse to a greater extent at the front, forming a wedge shape. When you pile several of these wedge-shaped vertebrae on top of one another, the spine bends forward and takes on a hunched appearance. The physical change in the back often causes the abdominal area to be compressed and bulge out. Not surprisingly, these changes in appearance can cause a loss of self-esteem. In another survey of women with vertebral abnormalities from osteoporosis, researchers from the University of Northern Colorado found that 19% of them were embarrassed at the appearance of their back and 21% said they had trouble finding clothes that fit properly.[10]

Importance of Family History and Genetics

The ability to build bone mass as a youngster and to hold onto it during aging is driven not only by lifestyle choices but by genetics as well. Just as you inherit a certain hair and eye color from your parents, you also inherit characteristics related to your bones. In addition to the direct influence of genetics on building and maintaining bone mass, your genes can influence other aspects of risks related to osteoporosis. Your eyesight, physical coordination, and "natural" ability to keep your balance are all important factors related to your risk of falling and thus incurring an osteoporotic fracture. Your family history, or inherited risk, to develop other medical or physical conditions that are seemingly unrelated to osteoporosis will also impact your risk of fracture. Conditions that require you to take medications that make you drowsy, cause you to lose your balance, or become dizzy can increase your likelihood of falling and fracturing.

The inheritance of bone mass is a topic that has caught the interest of researchers for several decades. Early studies used x-rays of the hand to measure the thickness of bones in the fingers of parents and their children. Following the introduction of more sophisticated instruments for measuring bone density, additional studies were done comparing bone density in parents and their children. By measuring the bone density in mother-daughter pairs, it's been estimated that 46% of our bone mass is a result of heredity.[11] Of course, both parents should have an influence on the bone density of their children. In fact, a stronger correlation is found when the bone density of both the father and mother are considered. In these studies, the parents' bone density accounted for 52% to 72% of the bone mass in their daughters.

A study published in the *New England Journal of Medicine* by researchers in Melbourne, Australia, examined the bone density of daughters who had mothers with osteoporosis and daughters with mothers who were osteoporosis-free.[12] Not surprisingly, they found lower bone density in the spines and hips of daughters with mothers who had osteoporosis. However, a more significant discovery was that the difference in bone density among the two groups of daughters was much less than the difference in bone density between the two groups of mothers. This means that lifestyle factors in adulthood may be at least as important, if not more important, than genetics when it comes to bone loss during aging. This study, and other similar studies of bone density among family members, have provided important insights to the effects of heredity on bone mass. In addition, within a family there are other important potential influences unrelated to genetics that account for the similarities in bone mass among family members. For example, some families may have hobbies or other interests that keep them more physically active. Food intake behaviors that determine calcium intake can vary widely among families. These habits and lifestyle practices are often "passed down" from parents and manifest themselves years later in the form of chronic diseases, or a lack of disease, in their children. These other "family factors" complicate the interpretation of genetic studies of bone mass within families.

The flaw in interpreting studies that attempt to determine hereditary influences on bone mass among family members became strikingly clear to me one day when two women approached me, following a lecture I gave on the importance of calcium nutrition for the prevention of osteoporosis. Although both women were obviously elderly, their physical appearances were remarkably different. The first woman was above average in height and had very straight posture and an overall robustness in her movements. The second woman was much shorter, walked with the assistance of a cane, and was quite frail-looking. To my surprise, the women told me they were twins. Based on their own personal experience, they knew how critically important calcium was for health. As it turned out, the two women had cultivated very different calcium intake habits throughout their lives. One had always liked milk and had consumed three to four glasses per day since childhood; the other, who never liked milk and never drank it, was suffering from severe osteoporosis. From this point on, it was very clear to me that studies of twins were the only viable way to really understand the relative importance of genetics versus environment on bone density.

Studies of bone mass in twins compare the difference between identical and fraternal pairs. Since identical twins share the exact same genetic code, differences in their bone mass are attributable to environmental influences. On the other hand, bone mass differences among fraternal twins will be the result of both genetic and environmental influences. By comparing the differences between these types of twin pairs, the percentage of bone mass determined by genetics can be measured. A number of these twin studies have been completed and clearly show a genetic influence on bone gain during growth and development. However, the influence of genetics on bone loss during aging is unclear at this time. The data we do have suggests that environmental factors are at least as important, if not more important, than genetics. This interpretation would be consistent with the study of mother-daughter pairs described earlier, in which bone mass was 33% different in osteoporotic women versus non-osteoporotic women, but only 7% different in their adult daughters.

From the twin studies, the influence of genetics on bone mass has been estimated at approximately 50% to 80%.[13–15] Even if we assume that the high estimate of 80% is correct, that leaves 20% of our total bone mass under environmental, or lifestyle, control. That may not seem like much, but let's look at it from a perspective that's easier to understand. Twin studies have also been conducted to determine the genetic influence on body height. Interestingly, about the same degree of genetic influence has been estimated for height as for bone mass, approximately 80%. Using myself as an example (I'm 6′ 2″), the 20% environmental influences equate to a difference of about seven inches either up or down—obviously a huge difference.

Of course, calcium, per se, has not been shown to increase height in well-nourished children. However, it has been shown to give children added bone density and, therefore, strength. Furthermore, the difference in bone density is similar in magnitude to the difference predicted by the genetic models. In the first and only study in the world to test the effects of added calcium on bone mass in identical twin children, preadolescent twin pairs were given either a placebo or CCM as the calcium source.[16–19] Although their calcium intake from diet alone already exceeded the RDA for calcium, the addition of CCM yielded bone density increases that were about 20% greater (you can read more about CCM supplement studies in children in Chapter 4). This study, which was published in the *New England Journal of Medicine* in 1992, clearly showed that calcium is an important environmental influence on bone density. Furthermore, it emphasizes the fact that regardless of whether we are genetically preprogrammed to have high, or low, bone density, there are lifestyle changes we can make to ensure we reach our genetic potential.

Lifestyle Factors That Impact Risk

Besides calcium intake, there are numerous other lifestyle factors that interact with your genetic makeup to determine skeletal health. The importance of some of the diet-related lifestyle factors have been greatly over-emphasized while others are greatly under-appreciated. What follows is a guide to understanding the most important factors for bone health in otherwise healthy people. There are other factors related to certain diseases or medical conditions that impact bone health directly or through medications used in their management.[5] You should be aware of these factors so that you can discuss them with your physician if it is appropriate. They include: (1) androgen deficiency (especially in men), which accelerates bone loss; (2) the use of corticosteroids, which can contribute to bone loss; (3) thyroid hormone replacement, which, if you're over-medicated, can increase bone loss; (4) diuretics, which, depending on the type of diuretic used, can either increase or decrease urinary output of calcium; and (5) rheumatoid arthritis, which seems to go hand in hand with the development of osteoporosis.

Physical Inactivity

In my view, physical activity is at least as important as calcium for maintaining lifelong skeletal health. The old adage "use it or lose it" clearly applies to bone. Bones respond to mechanical stresses placed on them. The flip side of this is that bone also responds to a lack of mechanical stress. The skeleton serves two main functions. First, it is a calcium reserve that can be called on when the body's calcium intake is too low. Since calcium is vital for the functioning of virtually every cell you have, your body will automatically pull calcium from its bones if you don't eat enough. The second function of the skeleton is to provide mechanical stability. Bones protect internal organs and give our muscles something to pull against so we can move.

Physical activity is at least as important as calcium for maintaining lifelong skeletal health. The old adage "use it or lose it" clearly applies to bone.

The mechanical stability function of bones is highly responsive to our environment. During times when the skeleton is "unloaded," or not experiencing stimulus telling it to be strong, it adapts by becoming weaker (i.e., bone loss occurs). The classic example of this unloading effect is the loss of calcium during space flight. The zero-gravity environment of space essentially removes any need for mechanical strength in the skeleton. When bone density, and therefore calcium, is lost, there's no place for the calcium to go except out through the urine. This is exactly what has been seen in studies of astronauts.[20] They experience a tremendous outpouring of calcium in their urine.

When it comes to unloading the skeleton, the closest thing to zero-gravity space flight on earth is bed rest. Although bed rest occurs at 1 G (gravity) force, body weight is spread out laterally across the entire skeleton, which substantially reduces the need for mechanical strength in the bones. A number of bed rest studies in healthy volunteers have shown that the rate of calcium loss under this circumstance equates to a 6% loss of bone density per year.[20]

The opposite of unloading the skeleton is to "load" the skeleton in such a way that greater than body weight force and/or greater than 1 G force is applied. This occurs with simple daily activities such as walking, climbing stairs, lifting, carrying, and, of course, with exercise. Unfortunately, it appears to be much easier to lose bone with disuse than to build bone with physical activity. Controlled studies of the effect of weight-bearing exercise programs have shown only modest gains in bone density.[21] In addition, as with other benefits of physical activity such as cardiovascular fitness, if you stop exercising you lose the benefit.[22]

Despite the somewhat less than impressive results shown in controlled studies of loading the skeleton, the positive benefits of regular physical activity on bone health measured in the population at large is quite impressive and consistent. A number of studies have shown that bone density is higher in children, adults, and older adults who are physically active. Moreover, hip fracture rates are *lower* in women with a history of physical activity.[22] This probably indicates the combined effects of physical activity on bone density, muscle strength, agility, and coordination, all of which lend added protection against falling and fracturing. The benefit of physical activity may be like the benefit of calcium, in that a lifelong strategy is needed to yield optimal results, but benefits can be obtained at any age.

Studies of active, as compared to sedentary, people have provided some interesting principles about the benefits of physical activity to the skeleton. First, increases in bone density only occur at the skeletal site or sites being stressed. A classic example of this is the observation that density is greater in the bones of your dominant arm. Taking this a step further, tennis players have significantly greater bone density in the forearm of their racket arm.[23,24] Besides the normal everyday use of the dominant arm, the racket arm undergoes significant shock and torque when the ball is hit. Another interesting example is that female figure skaters have greater bone density in their hips and legs compared to nonathletes.[25] Furthermore, bone density is greater in the hip and leg on the side they normally land on following a jump. The take-away message is, don't expect exercise with one part of the body to benefit bones at another skeletal site.

Another principle for applying the benefits of exercise to bone is that it must be "weight-bearing" exercise. You need to generate greater force on the bone than it normally experiences at rest from body weight alone. Walking is a mild form of weight-bearing exercise. Every time your heel and foot strike the ground, additional force is applied to the bones going from your foot up through your hip. Jogging, running, and jumping rope apply even greater forces. In fact, some health professionals recommended simply jumping up and down a few times a day to help keep bones in the lower body strong. Weight training is another way to apply above-normal force to the skeleton. Heavy (relative to the individual), basic movements with free weights (not machines) that use all the major muscle groups of the upper and lower body are probably best. A prime illustration of the need for a weight-bearing component in physical activity comes from studies done with swimmers. Swimming is an excellent exercise for improving cardiovascular fitness, muscle endurance, and strength throughout the whole body. However, it takes place in an essentially weightless environment. Thus, it's not surprising to find that swimmers, even elite-level competitors, have bone densities no greater than sedentary individuals.[22]

The final exercise principle to keep in mind is that too much of it may be harmful to your bones. High intensity sports participation, be it competitive or recreational, can be detrimental to your skeleton in several ways. For example, the below-normal body weight that often accompanies serious participation in long distance running can cause hormonal abnormalities. Studies with female athletes who have menstrual disturbances show they have lower bone densities than women with normal menses.[26,27] Estrogen levels drop in these women and they go through a quasi-menopause, including the expected negative effect on their bones. Even male long distance runners have been reported to have low spinal bone density.[28,29] Another problem related to exercise and your bones is stress fractures.[30,31] The repeated pounding of certain areas of the skeleton that comes with intense and regular practice of a single type of physical activity often leads to stress fractures, which are more common in athletes with lower bone density. This is one reason why it's better to "cross-train" or mix up the types of exercises you do. Not only does this reduce your chances of developing overuse-type injuries, but it keeps your exercise program more interesting, challenging, and complete. A final caution about exercise and skeletal health concerns the loss of calcium in sweat. It's not uncommon for serious athletes to produce one to two quarts—or more—of sweat a day, particularly when the weather is hot. Since the calcium content of sweat averages about 50 mg per quart, that means they must replace 50–100 mg per day.[32] Couple this with the facts that calcium is generally not well-absorbed and that some athletes shy away from dairy products, and you come up with a very undesirable set of circumstances for maintaining the health of bone.

If, for whatever reason, you are not ready, willing, or able to participate in some type of regular physical activity, take heart. Remember that disuse (unloading) seems to be a more potent cause of poor skeletal health than exercise is a positive driver for good bone health. Use your bones and muscles in simple, everyday opportunities. Take the stairs, take a walk, and don't drive around the parking lot for five minutes looking for the closest possible space. Find an activity you enjoy, or at least can tolerate, and make it a priority.

Smoking

A number of studies have shown that smokers have significantly lower bone densities than nonsmokers. This observation has been made mainly in older men and postmenopausal women who had a long history of smoking. However, at least one study has also shown that smoking during adolescence and young adulthood can reduce the gains in bone density that are usually made during this phase of life.[33] Depending on the age of the subjects, duration of smoking, and the part of the skeleton that is measured, bone mass differences between smokers and nonsmokers have been reported to be as great as 4%–22%.[34,35]

One of the longest and most interesting studies of the effect of smoking on bone mass was conducted with male identical twins.[14] Bone loss rates were measured over a 16-year period, comparing the smoking twin with his nonsmoking sibling (cotwin). Average bone loss rates were found to be 44% greater in the smoking twin. In addition, loss rates were linked to the quantity of cigarettes smoked—those who smoked more, lost more bone.

One of the most recent (1997) studies that reported on smoking and bone loss involved Japanese-American men living in Hawaii.[34] Bone loss rates were measured over a five-year period in three groups of men, with an average age of 68 years: current smokers, past smokers, and those who never smoked. Compared to the men who never smoked, rates of bone loss were 25% greater in smokers and 20% greater in past smokers. The duration and quantity of smoking also affected bone loss. Significantly greater rates of loss were seen in the men who smoked more than one pack of cigarettes per day and who had been smoking the longest. Based on the bone loss rates, the researchers estimated that fracture risk was increased 30% per decade of smoking.

Alcohol

There is no doubt that excessive alcohol consumption can lead to osteoporosis. The prevalence of alcoholism in postmenopausal women with hip or wrist fractures is almost four times greater than in women without fractures.[36] This probably reflects the combined effects of a greater risk of falling, poorer overall nutrition and health, and the direct effects of alcohol on bone or calcium metabolism. It also appears that fairly moderate alcohol consumption will contribute to greater losses of bone during aging when other factors are controlled. For example, in the study of male identical twins, bone loss rates were 41% greater in men consuming 1.5 drinks per day compared to the nondrinking group.[14] In addition, the effects of alcohol and smoking have a cumulative effect on bone loss. The men with the lowest bone-loss rates were nonsmokers and nondrinkers (the control group). Intermediate rates of bone loss (40%–45% higher than in the control group) occurred in men who either drank or smoked more than the average. The highest rates of bone loss (twice as great as the control group) were found in the group of men with both above-average alcohol consumption and above-average tobacco use.

Sodium

Sodium intake is one of the most often ignored nutritional factors related to calcium metabolism and bone health. Most people think of hypertension (high blood pressure) when it comes to issues of sodium and health. However, the data are very clear regarding sodium intake as an important risk factor for bone health as well. In fact, sodium may be as important as calcium. The relationship between sodium and calcium is via the effects of sodium on the urinary excretion of calcium.[37,38]

Although we are very efficient at absorbing sodium, our bodies have essentially no capacity to store extra sodium over the long run. Thus, essentially 100% of our sodium intake is absorbed and then excreted in the urine. Before sodium ends up in urine, it must be filtered from the blood by our kidneys. As the kidneys filter blood, both sodium and calcium are removed. However, since sodium and calcium are absolutely vital for normal cell function, the kidneys also work by reabsorbing both elements back into the bloodstream. This reabsorption pathway is where the sodium-calcium interaction takes place. A common pathway is used by the kidneys for both calcium and sodium. Thus, greater amounts of sodium compete with calcium and limit its reabsorption. The net effect of all this is: The more sodium you eat, the more calcium you excrete. This relationship has been shown in men, women, and children.

For each 57 mg of sodium you ingest, you lose about 1 mg of calcium.[38] That may not seem like very much, but let's run through some numbers to put the sodium effect into perspective. The upper limit of the recommended sodium intake for adults is 2,400 mg per day.[39] Note that this is not a recommended intake; rather, it is the upper limit of intake, above which health risks from excess sodium begin to rise. Typical intakes are much higher than this, averaging 4,000 mg in adult Americans. The high sodium intake in our country comes from the consumption of processed foods containing salt, the addition of salt to homecooked meals, and use of the salt shaker at the dinner table. On average, we exceed the upper limit of the recommended sodium intake by 1,600 mg per day. This excess sodium causes the excretion of an extra 28 mg of calcium per day. Over the course of a year, the loss of an extra 28 mg of calcium per day is equivalent to an annual 1% loss of total body calcium, a rate very similar to that experienced by postmenopausal women.

Researchers from Australia have recently completed a study of the relationship among calcium, sodium, and bone loss in postmenopausal women.[40] Like many other studies, this one showed that sodium intake was the major cause of urinary calcium excretion. In addition, the researchers documented a significant negative association between sodium intake and bone loss in the hip. The higher the sodium intake, the greater the amount of bone loss. They calculated that a sodium intake of 3,000 mg per day would require a calcium intake of 1,700 mg to offset bone loss. If sodium intake were brought down to the upper intake limit, then only 1,200 mg of calcium would be needed. These data show that a very high calcium intake can overcome the negative effect of high sodium intake. However, a more reasonable approach is to lower sodium intake, which allows for a more attainable level of calcium intake.

Protein

Unlike sodium, protein appears to be a double-edged sword when it comes to bone loss. On the one hand, low protein intake appears to be detrimental to bone density, especially in the elderly, who often have low protein intakes. Protein supplements have repeatedly been shown to have a beneficial effect on the healing of hip fractures.[41,42] On the other hand, a dietary excess of protein has clearly been shown to increase urinary calcium excretion. In a four-year prospective study of bone density in women in their 20s, the most important determinant of bone density change was the ratio of calcium to protein in the diet.[43] For every gram of protein intake, 1.5 mg of calcium is lost in the urine. Typically, postmenopausal women exceed the RDA for protein by about 10 grams per day.[39,44] This equates to an additional loss of 15 mg of calcium per day, which, on a yearly basis, represents a loss of 0.5% of total body calcium.

Caffeine

Reports of caffeine's negative effect on calcium and bone metabolism have been greatly overstated in the past. Initial reports focused on the effect of coffee consumption on the excretion of calcium in the urine during the immediate post-coffee consumption period. These early studies showed that coffee, or chemical pure caffeine, can raise urine calcium output. However, follow-up studies of longer duration demonstrated that caffeine causes an initial rise followed by a subsequent drop in urine calcium output. Thus, the net effect of caffeine is quite small and can be offset by the addition of two tablespoons of milk per cup of coffee.[2] Nevertheless, in the long run, small increases in urine calcium excretion can add up to significant losses in bone density. This led several research groups to investigate the relationship of caffeine intake to bone loss and fracture incidence in postmenopausal women. *Most of these studies failed to find any association between caffeine intake and bone health.* When a relationship was found, it seemed to apply only to women with dietary calcium intakes below 800 mg per day. Although this value is substantially below intake recommendations for postmenopausal women (1,200–1,500 mg per day), it is substantially higher than what they actually consume. Currently, only 20% of postmenopausal women consume 800 mg or more of calcium per day.[44]

A problem in interpreting many of the past studies of caffeine intake and bone density is the presence of confounding factors. For example, heavy coffee drinkers frequently smoke, and tobacco use is known to accelerate bone loss rates. In addition, several previous caffeine studies did not control for hormone replacement therapy, which has a major impact on bone density. Furthermore, caffeine intakes in these studies were estimated rather than actually measured. People vary widely in how they prepare coffee or tea at home or work. This leads to caffeine levels in the same volume of coffee or tea that may vary by three- to fivefold.

To address these problems in study design, researchers in the College of Medicine at Penn State University conducted an experiment in which great care was taken to isolate the effect of caffeine on bone density in postmenopausal women. The study was published in 1997 in the *American Journal of Clinical Nutrition* and represents the latest findings in caffeine research.[45] To make an accurate assessment of caffeine intake, samples of the caffeine-containing beverages consumed by the study subjects were collected and chemically analyzed. In addition, a wide range of confounding variables, such as smoking and hormone replacement therapy, were used to exclude subjects from participating. Three groups of women were recruited, based on their usual caffeine intake: low caffeine users (zero to two cups of coffee per day), moderate users (three to four cups per day), and high users (five or more cups per day). No significant differences in bone density of the hip or total body were found in the three groups. Moreover, when all the women were combined to form a single group with coffee and/or tea consumption ranging from zero cups to eight cups per day, no significant relationship was found between caffeine intake and bone density. Finally, even when low-calcium consumers (500 mg per day) were examined, no significant effect of caffeine on bone density was found.

Estrogen Therapy

The issue of whether to use estrogen replacement therapy is something every woman reaching menopause must face. It's a somewhat complicated, and sometimes frightening, decision that should only be made after thorough discussions with your doctor regarding your own personal risk factors and the potential benefits and disadvantages. Hormone replacement therapy can reduce the typical symptoms of menopause such as hot flashes, vaginal dryness, and mood swings. In addition, and more importantly for long-term health, estrogen therapy can significantly reduce your risk (by about 50%) for coronary artery disease, which typically becomes a greater threat to women following menopause. Estrogen's benefits for a healthy circulatory system apparently come from its positive actions on blood cholesterol levels and direct effects on the walls of the arteries.

Estrogen stops the bone loss that occurs at the time of menopause and may actually cause a slight increase in bone density. It has also been shown to provide a fracture protection benefit. However, the benefits of estrogen on preventing fractures are dependent on when estrogen is started and how long it is used.[46] Estrogen is most protective against fractures if started early and used for more than 10 years. For example, peripheral fracture risk is reduced by 50% in current long-term estrogen users who started within five years of menopause. However, the fracture protection benefits are substantially reduced if estrogen is initiated more than five years after menopause. Also, the protective effect of estrogen diminishes once estrogen is stopped, so that previous usage does not necessarily convey a long-term benefit.

Although calcium and other lifestyle factors can have a major impact on the bone loss process, they cannot substitute for estrogen. The reason is quite simple. Estrogen, calcium, and physical activity all protect against bone loss. However, at menopause, women become estrogen-deficient independent of their calcium intake, level of physical activity, or any other factor. As such, estrogen deficiency can only be corrected by replacing estrogen.[47] Of course, optimizing your calcium and physical activity habits will go a long way toward keeping your skeleton healthy. In fact, as you will read in the following section, the addition of calcium to estrogen replacement therapy greatly enhances its effectiveness. Nevertheless, the point still stands, nothing can correct an estrogen deficiency except estrogen.

The negative side of the risk-benefit equation for estrogen primarily centers around concerns about cancer. The risk of endometrial cancer is up to six times greater in women with an intact uterus receiving unopposed estrogen therapy (estrogen without progestin). This risk is removed when estrogen-progestin combinations are used. For breast cancer, a number of studies have indicated that estrogen replacement therapy, or combined estrogen-progestin therapy, significantly increases risk. In addition, the older you are and the longer you take hormone replacement therapy, the greater the risk. A large study recently published in the *New England Journal of Medicine* showed that a usage period of less than five years appears to have borderline effects on breast cancer risk. However, women ages 55 to 59 who used hormones for at least five years have about a 50% greater risk and those 60 to 64 years with five years or more of hormone usage have a 70% increase in risk.[48] Thus, estrogen therapy is contraindicated for women known to have breast cancer, a past experience with breast cancer, or a strong family history of breast cancer. Since new information is always being gathered regarding the risks and benefits of estrogen replacement therapy, the best thing to do is thoroughly discuss the issue with your physician. If you can't get the level of information that makes you comfortable with your decision, then consult other physicians until you're satisfied.

How to Triple the Effect of Estrogen with Calcium

As you will repeatedly read in various sections of this book, calcium is the basic building block of bone. No matter what else you do to promote a healthy skeleton, you've got to have calcium. You can't build a house without the lumber. This fundamental need for calcium extends to drug treatments for bone as well. Concomitant calcium supplementation or modifying one's diet to a higher calcium intake should always be part of any prescription therapy for osteoporosis. The value of this combined approach, double therapy if you will, was made quite clear by a recent study (1998) from researchers at the Helen Hayes Hospital and Columbia University.[49] They reviewed the published literature on the effect of estrogen therapy on bone mass with or without calcium. The results for calcium were truly outstanding.

No matter what else you do to promote a healthy skeleton, you've got to have calcium. You can't build a house without the lumber.

Thirty-one separate studies were used in the analysis. The average length of the studies was about 2.5 years. In 11 of the studies, estrogen was given with no modification to calcium intake. The women in these estrogen-only studies had an average calcium intake of 563 mg per day, which is very close to the average calcium intake by all postmenopausal women living in America.[44] Twenty of the studies used the double therapy of estrogen plus calcium by giving supplements or by modifying the diet. The average calcium intake of the women in these studies was 1,183 mg per day, a value close to, but slightly below, the current range of recommended calcium intakes for postmenopausal women of 1,200–1,500 mg per day.[2,50] In the women treated with estrogen alone, bone mass change averaged +0.87%. However, the women receiving estrogen plus calcium had an average bone mass change of +2.6%, a threefold increase in the effect. The results were consistent across skeletal sites. In the spine, calcium increased the estrogen effect on bone mass from +1.3% (estrogen alone) to +3.3% (estrogen plus calcium). In the hip, the effect went from about +1.0% up to +2.5%. In the forearm, calcium increased the estrogen effect from about +0.5% to +2.0%.

CHAPTER FOUR

CCM and Bone Building in Children

- Superior Calcium Absorption from CCM in Children
- The Importance of Peak Bone Mass
- CCM and Bone Building in Young Children
- CCM and Bone Building in Teenagers
- How High Is Up? CCM Goes to Summer Camp
- Bone Mass and Fractures in Children

Clinical studies of the effectiveness of CCM have been on the leading edge of calcium research in children for the last 10 years. Besides documenting nutritional benefits of CCM, this work produced some of the first information on true calcium absorption in children.[1,2] In addition, it provided the very first direct evidence that bone building in children could be increased with extra calcium even if their diets already met recommended intake standards.[3] Because this work with CCM led to landmark findings in the field of calcium nutrition in general, it has been very influential in reshaping the thinking about optimal calcium intake during childhood and adolescence. Indeed, the information on the effects of CCM has been used extensively by the National Institutes of Health and the National Academy of Sciences in setting and revising recommendations for calcium intake in children.[4,5]

Bone building in childhood and adolescence is equally, if not more, important than reducing bone loss during aging.

The most effective way to reduce the lifetime risk of developing osteoporosis is to use a two-step approach. The first step is maximizing bone building during the growth and development years. The second step is maintaining bone mass as an adult by minimizing loss of bone. Until recently, the first part of this equation for lifelong bone health had been largely ignored. However, it is now becoming widely recognized that bone building in childhood and adolescence is equally, if not more, important than reducing bone loss during aging. In addition, building greater bone density when we're young not only provides protection against fractures later in life but yields an immediate protection benefit against fractures during childhood.

Superior Calcium Absorption from CCM in Children

Optimizing peak bone mass development during growth and development in childhood is universally recognized as one of the most important things we can do to lower our lifetime risk for osteoporosis. In fact, according to the National Academy of Sciences, *the most* important nutritional approach for reducing osteoporosis in our society is to ensure a calcium intake that allows children to reach their genetic potential for building bone mass.[6] Achieving the calcium intake during childhood and adolescence that optimizes peak bone mass is a multi-step process. First, the right choices of calcium-rich foods must be made. This includes foods that are naturally high in calcium, as well as foods that have been fortified with calcium. When needed, calcium supplements for kids and adolescents are a viable approach for augmenting the calcium level in the diet up to the optimal amount.

For many children, a combination of all three approaches (foods, fortified foods, and supplements) will be needed to obtain a consistent intake at recommended levels. This phase of life is too critical to lifelong bone health not to use all the tools available for boosting calcium intake. Remember, about 95% of the skeleton's maximum size and weight, or peak bone mass, is built by 18 years of age (see Figure 4-1).[7] Moreover, during puberty, kids build about 50% of their peak bone mass.

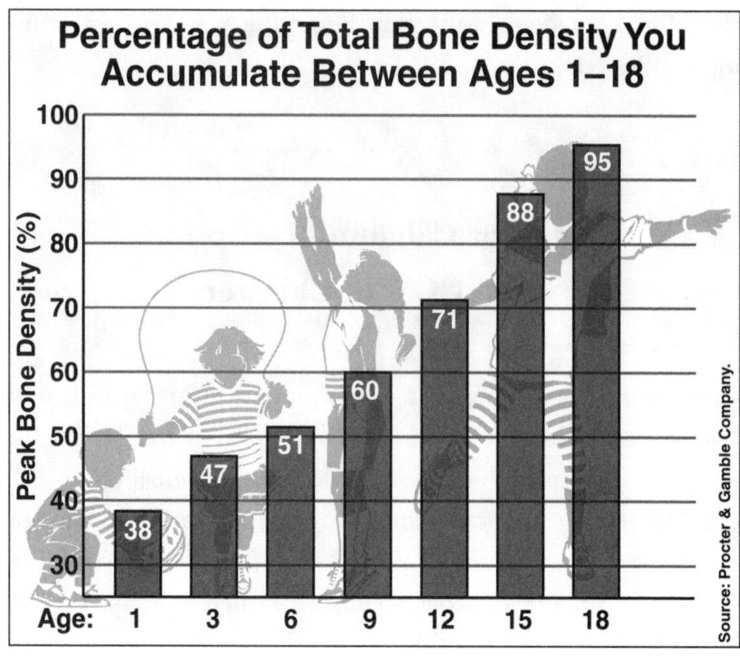

Figure 4-1

By the time you turn 18 years old,
you've built 95% of your peak bone mass.

Calcium intake, per se, is the foundation for ensuring the optimization of peak bone mass development. However, it's only part of the equation. To benefit the skeleton, the calcium that is consumed needs to absorbed. Once it is absorbed and used to develop the skeleton, younger kids and adolescents should pursue the lifestyle behaviors that help the skeleton retain its calcium and minimize those factors that draw calcium out of the bone. For the most part, these lifestyle factors are the same for kids and adults. The positive ones include a well-balanced diet with optimal amounts of calcium and other nutrients, and exercise, especially weight-bearing exercise. Negative factors are a sedentary lifestyle, too high of a sodium intake, tobacco, and alcohol.

For many years it was believed that children had a much greater ability to absorb calcium than adults. This belief was partially based on intuition. That is, since kids are actively building their skeletons, and calcium is needed for bone growth, then nature will provide a way for kids to absorb greater amounts of calcium during periods of rapid growth. But the belief was also based on studies of laboratory animals, in which it was fairly easy to demonstrate a dramatic difference in calcium absorption among weanling, juvenile, and adult animals.[8]

We now know that calcium absorption is actually very similar in kids and adults. Kids may, in fact, have a slight advantage in absorption ability, but it's not nearly as great as once was thought. This is a critical point in determining the right calcium intake recommendation for children. If they are less efficient at absorbing calcium than was previously estimated, then a greater intake is needed. Some of the first direct evidence of calcium absorption in children came from studying CCM in healthy adolescent girls and boys. This was a collaborative study among the Procter & Gamble Company, the Department of Medicine at Indiana University, and the Department of Medicinal Chemistry at Purdue University. It was funded by the National Institutes of Health and Procter & Gamble.[1]

Six healthy boys and six healthy girls between the ages of 10 and 17 agreed to participate in the study. Permission was also obtained from their parents. To ensure that they were healthy, all the children had a medical exam, which included a physical exam, medical history, and routine laboratory tests of blood and urine. Calcium absorption was measured twice in each child, once using CCM as the calcium source, and the second time using calcium carbonate. Calcium carbonate is the most common supplemental source of calcium and has been shown in a number of studies to provide calcium that is as well-absorbed as the calcium in milk and a number of other calcium sources including calcium citrate, calcium lactate, and calcium gluconate.[9–11]

Your body can't make calcium; you must take it from the environment to build and maintain a healthy skeleton.

Since calcium absorption was measured from both CCM and calcium carbonate, each child was able to serve as his or her own control. In this way, a very accurate comparison could be made between the two calcium sources. Another important aspect of this study was that the test sources of calcium were given to the children along with a meal. This was done to more accurately mimic a real-life situation, where calcium is normally consumed along with other foods as part of a meal.

The results from the study showed that calcium absorption averaged 36% when the children were given CCM but only 26% when they were given calcium carbonate. This represents a 37% increase in calcium absorption of CCM over calcium carbonate. In addition to the significant rise in calcium absorption from CCM, another interesting observation was made. The calcium absorption values found in the children were very close to those obtained when adults were studied. Calcium absorptions from CCM and calcium carbonate in children were compared in a second study funded by the National Institutes of Health.[2] A similar study protocol was utilized, but this time two different CCM preparations were used. The study showed that the two CCM preparations did not differ in terms of calcium absorption and averaged 41%. Calcium absorption from calcium carbonate was again shown to be significantly lower, at only 27%. *This represented a calcium absorption advantage by CCM of 52% over calcium carbonate.*

Another study recently completed by researchers at the U.S. Department of Agriculture's Children's Nutrition Research Center and the Department of Pediatrics at Baylor College of Medicine also shows that children and adults are very close in terms of their calcium absorption abilities.[12] Calcium absorption was measured in 12 children (7 boys, 5 girls) using milk and spinach as the calcium sources. The researchers reported 27% calcium absorption from milk and only 3% from spinach. These values resemble those reported in a similar study conducted on adults. In the adult study, 13 subjects consumed calcium as milk or spinach along with a standard meal. Absorption was found to be 28% from milk and only 5% from spinach.[13]

In addition to showing the similarities between adults and children for calcium absorption, all of these studies taken together show the dramatic range of calcium absorption that can be obtained from common food sources. Calcium from spinach is hardly absorbed at all, milk and calcium carbonate show absorptions in the middle to high 20s, and CCM yields a high calcium absorption in the middle 30s to lower 40s.

The Importance of Peak Bone Mass

Your body can't make calcium; you must take it from the environment to build and maintain a healthy skeleton. As a fetus develops in the womb, calcium is supplied by the mother. Very little calcium accumulates until the last trimester of pregnancy, and even then, the baby's amount of bone mineralization is quite low. In utero, there is no advantage to building a strong skeletal framework. As a fetus, we are suspended in an essentially weightless environment and have no need for mechanically strong bones. In fact, a rigid skeleton would be quite counter-productive to the birthing process.

When we begin our ex-utero life, our supply of calcium switches from the maternal blood supply to the food we eat. As a full-term newborn infant, we start off with about 25 grams of calcium in our total body. By the time our skeleton reaches its maximum size and weight, this value will have increased to about 1,300 grams for an average-sized man and 1,000 grams for the average women. This maximum size and weight of the skeleton is known as peak bone mass.

The importance of peak bone mass and how it relates to our lifetime risk of osteoporosis is a concept that has come of age during the last decade. For many years, the only emphasis placed on bone health for the population at large related to postmenopausal women with osteoporotic fractures and their need for medical management. We now realize that an osteoporotic fracture is simply one end of a continuum of bone health that begins early in life. The nutrition research community in particular has come to embrace the notion of optimizing peak bone mass as the single most important nutritional strategy for reducing the incidence of osteoporosis. Evidence for this can be seen in numerous publications that highlight this approach as the primary prevention strategy of choice. This is not to say that we are ever too old to benefit from optimizing calcium and other nutrient intakes for bone health. *In fact, a recent study (1997) showed that the number of fractures occurring in women and men ages 65 years and older could be reduced by over 50% by using CCM combined with vitamin D.*[14] However, we are never too young to start reaping the benefits of optimal calcium intake for lifelong skeletal health.

We are never too young to start reaping the benefits of optimal calcium intake for lifelong skeletal health. . . . A 5% greater peak bone mass in early life has been calculated to translate to a 50% or greater reduction in fractures later in life.

Using the analogy of saving money for your retirement years, you know that the earlier you start building your retirement nest egg, the larger it's going to be. So it is with bone health. The sooner you start making deposits to the bone bank, and the bigger those deposits are, the larger your account will be when you need it. Another concept related to this, which is equally important, is that small differences in the bone bank account pay large dividends. A 5% greater peak bone mass in early life has been calculated to translate to a 50% or greater reduction in fractures later in life.[3, 15–17]

Studying the Calcium–Bone Mass Relationship

Velimir Matkovic, M.D., Ph.D., was the first to observe the potential relationship between calcium intake early in life, peak bone mass formation, and fracture reduction in later life.[16] His seminal piece of work (published in 1979) kicked off an interest in calcium intake and peak bone mass that provided the foundation for other researchers to build on. In his study, Dr. Matkovic compared the bone mass and hip fracture rates of both men and women from two regions of the former Yugoslavia (now Croatia). One region was a "high" calcium-consuming area, with intakes that averaged about 1,000 mg per day. The other region, a "low" calcium-consuming area, had intakes of about 500 mg per day. A comparison of the bone mass measurements between inhabitants of the regions showed two things: First, the high calcium-consuming region had an average bone mass 6% greater than the low calcium-consuming region. Second, the difference in bone mass between the regions was already present at 30 years of age, the age of the youngest participants in the study. In other words, even though children and young adults were not actually studied, the fact that the bone mass difference was seen in adults showed that it had developed sometime before adulthood. In addition to calcium intake and bone mass, the hip fracture rates were dramatically different in the two regions. Men and women (ages 75+ years) from the low-calcium district had a fracture rate 3.5 to 4 times greater than those from the high-calcium district.

About a decade later a similar study (absent any fracture information) was conducted on people ages 35 years or older living in rural districts of China.[18] The districts were selected because the inhabitants' calcium intake was known to vary. In this case, the intake of the "high" calcium district was about 700 mg per day, and in the "low" calcium district, it averaged about 300 mg per day. Significant differences in bone density were observed between the high and low calcium-consuming districts. Also, the difference was present, and actually more pronounced, in the younger subject groups (ages 35 to 45). This study provided additional support for the idea that adult bone mass is strongly impacted by calcium intake during growth and development. However, direct evidence showing the relationship between calcium intake in childhood and bone density gains was still lacking.

To further explore this question, researchers in the United States took a different approach. A team from the University of Pittsburgh measured the bone mass in a group of postmenopausal women and then retrospectively measured their calcium intake during childhood.[19] This was done by asking the participants to remember back to meal times as a child and classify themselves as either always, sometimes, or rarely drinking milk with meals. They were asked to do this for childhood, adolescence, early adulthood, and later adulthood. In addition, the subjects completed a comprehensive evaluation of their current diet. No significant relationship was found between their current calcium intake and bone density. However, a significant relationship was found between their current bone density and their reported calcium intake in the past.

Bone density was about 3% greater in those who said they always drank milk with every meal during childhood and adolescence compared to those who said they rarely did. This value increased to almost 4% if the drinking of milk with every meal continued into early adulthood.

A similar study was conducted by a research team from the University of North Carolina except that instead of postmenopausal women, they studied premenopausal women with an average age of 35 years.[20] Again, bone density measurements were taken, information was collected about their current diets, and the subjects were asked to remember their past dairy product consumption habits from adolescence up to the present. From this, a lifetime calcium intake profile was developed for each subject and they were classified as either low, intermediate, or high lifetime calcium-consumers. In this case, low was defined as less 500 mg per day, intermediate was 500–800 mg per day, and high was greater than 800 mg per day. Bone density in the low calcium intake group was about 9% less than the intermediate and high lifetime calcium intake groups.

These studies formed the basis for emphasizing high calcium intake and bone building during childhood and adolescence as a way to increase fracture protection in adults. Although the information was compelling on its own, there were two outstanding issues that needed to be addressed. First, although it was clear from the studies with adults that peak bone mass was reached no later than age 30 or so, no one really knew how early bone density peaked. This was a critical issue to resolve because it would define the window of opportunity during which increased calcium would be effective for enhancing bone building. A number of studies were done to define the timing of peak bone mass in children. Unfortunately, just as the studies with adults had not gone low enough in age, the studies with children did not go high enough in age to define when the peak occurred.

If you are a premenopausal woman, even if you're in your late teens or early 20s, don't think of bone loss as something that's going to happen sometime in the future; it's already begun.

To find the exact timing of peak bone mass, a collaborative study between Ohio State University, Creighton University, and the Procter & Gamble Company was undertaken.[7] The key objective in this study was to determine the range of ages when peak bone mass occurred. Thus, bone mass in the whole skeleton and several individual skeletal sites was measured in females ranging in age from 8–50 years. The results showed that peak bone mass occurred in the mid-teens to early 20s, depending on skeletal site. An additional important discovery was that bone loss started at some skeletal sites immediately after the peak was reached. This debunked the long-held theory that once a woman reached her peak in bone mass, no bone loss occurred until menopause. Alarmingly, the two sites that showed a peak and then an immediate decline before the age of 20 years were the spine and hip. The loss of bone is slow at this time, slower than the typical loss experienced after menopause. Nevertheless, loss of bone density before menopause increases the risk of fracture after menopause and emphasizes the need for even very young adult women to maintain optimal calcium intake. If you are a premenopausal woman, even if you're in your late teens or early 20s, don't think of bone loss as something that's going to happen sometime in the future; it's already begun.

Besides the timing of peak bone mass, the second big issue that had to be addressed was the lack of direct evidence showing that increased calcium intake during childhood and adolescence was a cause of bone mass gain. The studies from Croatia, China, and the United States simply implied the relationship but didn't actually show it. Recall that the researchers concluded from these studies that calcium's benefit was manifesting itself during childhood. However, what the studies actually measured was calcium intake and bone mass in adults, not children. Even the retrospective studies were flawed in the way that information about childhood calcium intake was collected, because they relied on the subjects' 30- to 50-year-old memories. Sometimes I personally can't remember what I ate yesterday, let alone what I ate 30 years ago. The last, and perhaps most important, problem with these previous studies, is that they did not address the issue of optimal calcium intake. Groups with "low" calcium intakes in the 300 to 500 mg per day range (clearly inadequate) were compared to groups with "high" intakes in the 700 to 1,000 mg of calcium per day range. The breakthrough in understanding for optimal calcium intake and bone building in kids would come from studies with CCM.[3,21–35] In these studies, our "low" calcium intake groups picked up where the previous studies had left off, starting at 900 to 1,000 mg per day and going up from there.

CCM and Bone Building in Young Children

The very first study that attempted to directly demonstrate the importance of calcium to bone building in children was done with CCM. It was a collaborative study between the Departments of Medicine and Molecular Genetics at Indiana University and the Procter & Gamble Company. Funded by the National Institutes of Health and Procter & Gamble, this was the first study to directly show calcium's benefit to skeletal growth in children and was published in the *New England Journal of Medicine* in 1992.[3]

This study with CCM was unique in the field of calcium supplementation, in that it involved identical twin children. For three years, one twin within each pair was randomly assigned to receive an additional 1,000 mg of calcium per day supplied in the form of CCM. The other twin received an identical-looking placebo. Neither the children and their families nor the study investigators knew which twins were taking CCM. During the study, the children and their parents received no special instructions regarding what to eat. They just kept consuming their normal diets with the addition of either CCM or the placebo.

The use of identical twin children as subjects provided several other advantages for isolating the effect of CCM on bone building. First, all twin pairs were verified to be identical using blood tests. This means that within each pair, both children had the same genetic potential for skeletal growth and acquisition of bone mass. Second, identical twins, especially when they're young, tend to have environments that are more closely matched than non-twin siblings. They wear the same clothes, share the same bedroom, and their diets tend to be the same; if one plays soccer, the other usually plays, too. This combination of exactly matched genetics and very closely matched environmental conditions allowed us to, in essence, conduct the perfectly controlled study (or as near to perfect as you can get). However, the controlled nature of this study was not left to chance alone. A great deal of information about these children was gathered during the study to make sure that any differences in how they built bone could be accounted for and related back to CCM supplementation. For example, the diets the children consumed were very closely studied. In fact, the amount of data collected was greater than in any previous dietary study in children.

The average age of the preadolescent children who participated was seven years and both male and female twin pairs were involved. As was expected, during the three years of the study, there were no differences within each twin pair for height, weight, level of physical activity, or intake of nutrients from their diets. These children were healthy and very well-nourished. In fact, the calcium intake from diet alone (not including the CCM supplement) averaged 900 mg per day. This value actually exceeds the current recommended intake of calcium for this age group of 800 mg per day and makes the findings for CCM supplementation much more remarkable. The amount of extra calcium the CCM-supplemented group actually took was 700 mg per day, bringing their total calcium intake (diet plus CCM calcium) to 1,600 mg per day.

Bone density was measured at six different skeletal sites, and both groups gained bone density during the study. This is what you would expect to find for well-nourished growing children. However, at every bone site, the average increase was greater in the twin receiving CCM. In those who got the placebo, bone density increased about 15% in three years. *The bone density gain in the CCM group was 18% and represented a 20% greater rate of bone density acquisition. This increase in bone density, if maintained throughout adulthood, would be predicted to reduce lifetime fracture risk by 40% to 50%.*

Another important aspect of this work is that it called into question the adequacy of the recommended intake of calcium for children. Remember, the group that only got the placebo had a calcium intake from diet alone, which was somewhat *above* the recommended level. Yet the addition of more calcium in the form of CCM resulted in significantly greater gains in bone density.

CCM and Bone Building in Teenagers

Enhancing bone density gain in teenagers is perhaps even more important than for younger kids because of the rapid bone growth that occurs during puberty. About 50% of the peak adult bone mass you will ever develop is built during puberty. Although studies to directly test the benefit of calcium for bone building during puberty had not been conducted prior to the studies with CCM, scientists had long recognized that calcium needs were elevated during this phase of life. In 1997, the recommended intake for calcium during the teenage years was raised, due, in large part, to the studies conducted with CCM. Currently, compared to preadolescent children, the recommended amount of calcium during adolescence is 67% greater.[5] Unfortunately, this time of life is typically characterized by a decline in calcium intake. Just as their need for calcium increases, teenagers' intakes decrease. About 70% of teenage boys and 95% of teenage girls get less than the recommended amount of calcium.[5,36]

As with the CCM study of twins, the Penn State Young Women's Health Study was the first time that calcium was directly shown to benefit bone building in teenagers, in a double-blind, placebo-controlled experiment.[22] Penn State University and the Procter & Gamble Company combined their efforts and conducted the study at the Milton S. Hershey Medical Center, in Hershey, Pennsylvania. It was funded by the National Institutes of Health and Procter & Gamble. Normal healthy girls, just entering puberty, were recruited by working with the local school districts.

At random, one-half of the girls were assigned to receive 500 mg of extra calcium per day, provided in the form of CCM. The other half received an identical-looking placebo. Neither the subjects nor the research team knew who was getting CCM or the placebo. The girls continued to eat their usual diet and participate in whatever activities they chose. Dietary records were collected at regular intervals throughout the study to document how much calcium each group consumed from diet alone. There was no significant difference in calcium intake from diet in the two groups and the average intake was 960 mg per day.

In addition to the dietary information, many clinical measurements were collected during the study, especially those related to the expected hormonal changes of puberty. A unique feature of this study pertained to how bone density was measured. Just prior to initiating the study, a new and powerful tool for assessing bone density became available. We were fortunate to be the first group to put it to use in a double-blind, placebo-controlled study of calcium supplementation and bone density. This new technology, dual energy x-ray absorptiometry (DXA for short), was a critical leap in medical instrumentation for measuring bone health. It's now commonly used in many parts of the world, and if you have your bone density measured, it will most likely be with a DXA instrument. DXA is safe and painless, can be used repeatedly with children, and, most importantly for our study of teenage girls, allows for the measurement of bone density in the total skeleton. This technology was not yet available when the CCM and identical twins study was conducted. Consequently, measurements of bone density in that study relied on bone scans of small select areas of the skeleton. In contrast, the discovery of DXA permitted bone density of the total body to be measured, literally from head to foot. This is a very attractive scientific tool to use for studies of children because of our interest in their overall skeletal growth.

For an 18-month period, the girls supplemented their normal diets with either CCM or a placebo and had bone density measurements of the total body taken every six months. Both groups of girls grew normally throughout the study. There were no differences in their gains of height, weight, hormonal levels, or progression through puberty. However, there were very significant differences in the amount of bone density they added during the study (see Figure 4-2). *Although both groups gained bone density, as would be expected for growing teenagers, the girls receiving CCM gained at a significantly greater rate, about 20% more.*

Because bone density measurements were made every six months, it was possible to track the changes between the two groups as the study progressed. This analysis showed that bone density was already different between the two groups after just six months of CCM supplementation, and the two groups grew further and further apart as the study went on. Careful attention was also paid to documenting how much additional calcium they took from CCM. From this, we were able to determine that the additional bone density gains were achieved from the addition of

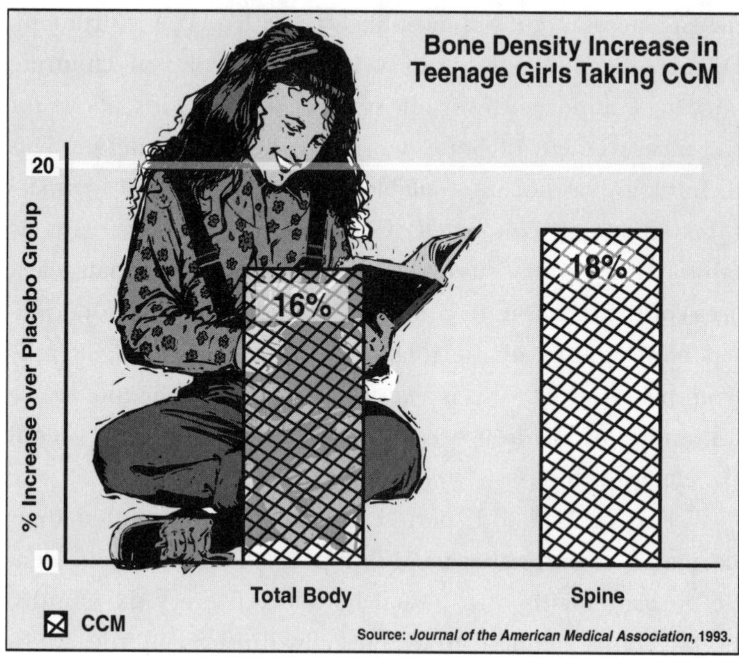

Figure 4-2

Teenage girls taking CCM gained 18% more bone density in the spine and 16% more in the total body than girls taking a placebo.

just 350 mg of extra calcium per day as CCM supplements. These results were submitted and accepted by the *Journal of the American Medical Association* (JAMA) and published in August 1993.

The study of teenage girls continued after the initial 18-month period to see if increased benefits from calcium supplementation in the form of CCM could be accomplished. The same groups of girls continued to take CCM or the placebo, and information about their diets, overall growth, and hormonal changes during puberty were collected. After two years of participating in the study, the girls were about 14 years of age. Bone density of the total body in the two groups continued to diverge, with the CCM group outpacing the placebo group. In addition, bone density measurements in the spine and pelvis showed that those girls receiving CCM were making 20%–22% greater gains compared to the placebo group.[35]

At this point, we faced an important decision regarding how best to continue the study. Although it was going well, we began to question what additional knowledge would be gained by continuing. The effect of CCM had been clearly demonstrated and was likely to continue the longer the study ran. The decision was made to petition the National Institutes of Health to allow a major change in the protocol. Since they were providing most of the funding for the study, their permission was required before any changes could be made. We proposed to discontinue CCM supplementation in one-half of the girls who had been taking it and start CCM supplementation in one-half of the girls who had been receiving the placebo. In this way, four study groups could be formed. One group would receive CCM for a total of four years; another would receive the placebo for four years. The other two groups would be supplemented with CCM for two years: One would take it early in puberty, and the other would begin taking it later in puberty. The National Institutes of Health approved the proposal and the protocol was changed.

As before, the girls, irrespective of their assignment to CCM or the placebo, made the expected gains in body size, hormonal progression, and bone density. However, the gains in bone density differed by treatment group. Following four years of treatment, the smallest increase in total body bone density occurred in the group who always received the placebo and only got calcium from their normal diet, which averaged about 900 to 1,000 mg of calcium per day. The greatest gains were observed for the group who had always been supplemented with CCM.[33] They averaged about 14% more bone density relative to the placebo group. The remaining two groups had bone density gains that were intermediate. These groups took CCM for only two years—one group for the first two years of the study, and the other for the second two years. These findings showed that CCM supplementation throughout puberty gives the best response. However, bone density benefits can also be made by supplementing either early or late in puberty.

From the study with teenage girls from the Hershey, Pennsylvania, area *it was clear that CCM supplementation, even at fairly modest levels, provided a benefit to bone density above and beyond that of calcium levels from the normal self-selected diet.* However, we wondered if this was the best we could do. Had we defined the optimal level of calcium for building peak bone mass? The answer, simply put, was no. By only using one level of supplementation, and a fairly low level at that (only 350 mg of calcium in the form of CCM), it was not possible to determine whether greater gains in bone density could be made. As such, a study was done to better define the ceiling for the bone building impact of CCM by using two levels of supplementation.[21]

As before, healthy, adolescent girls, just entering puberty, agreed to participate in a study of CCM supplementation and bone building. In addition to their normal diet, one group got a placebo, another received a medium amount of extra calcium in the form of CCM, and the third group got a higher amount of extra calcium as CCM. Average daily calcium intake during the six months the study lasted was about 900 mg for the placebo group (diet calcium only); 1,300 mg in the medium level CCM group (diet plus supplementation); and 1,600 mg in the group with a higher level of CCM (diet plus supplementation). Gains in total body bone mass were measured with DXA, and they mirrored the increases in calcium intake from CCM. The placebo group gained the least bone mass, whereas bone mass gains in the medium and higher CCM-supplemented groups were 10% and 23% greater, respectively. Since increasing levels of CCM supplementation were accompanied by increasing improvements in bone mass gain, with no hint that the effect was leveling off, we were not successful in defining the optimum calcium intake for maximizing bone building. However, with this additional work, we were able to show that increasing intakes up to 1,600 mg per day with CCM, which is about two times the normal calcium intake of a teenage girl, can provide significant benefits.

How High Is Up? CCM Goes to Summer Camp

The previous studies of adolescent females showed a very clear benefit to bone via the addition of CCM to the diet. Bone density and bone mass were increased by supplementing the diet with CCM up to a total calcium intake (diet plus CCM) between 1,300 and 1,600 mg per day. Even though these studies provided compelling evidence for increasing calcium intake during this important phase of life, researchers at Purdue University recognized, as did we, that the intake of calcium that would maximize peak bone mass development still eluded us. Part of the problem was that continuing to run long-term, placebo-controlled, double-blind studies with an ever increasing number of supplemented groups in order to find the ceiling for the bone building effect was too expensive to be practical. Consequently, the Purdue University research team chose to take a different approach, which would allow them to test multiple calcium intake levels of CCM in a period of weeks instead of months or years.[24]

The Purdue group dubbed their experiment "Camp Calcium" because the subjects who participated stayed on the Purdue University campus during the summer months in an environment created to mimic a typical summer camp atmosphere. This included staying in a sorority house and daily participation in various educational and recreational activities. At the same time, the diet of the study participants and, therefore, their calcium intake, were strictly controlled to the nearest tenth of a gram.

Adolescent girls were recruited from local school districts and they, along with their parents, agreed to participate in the study. All the girls were healthy, had a calcium intake from their normal diet of at least 800 mg per day, and were between the ages of 12 and 15. Two 21-day study periods were conducted, with a 4-week break in between. During the study periods, all of the foods and beverages the girls consumed were provided by the research team. The basic diet contained 800 mg of calcium and consisted of normal foods divided into three meals and two snacks per day. In addition to the basic diet, the girls consumed beverages that had been fortified with different amounts of CCM. The CCM beverages added extra calcium to their diets in amounts ranging from 41–1,373 mg per day. Thus, combined with the basic diet of 800 mg of calcium, their total intake of calcium ranged from 841–2,173 mg per day.

The benefit of calcium was measured using a technique that nutritionists call the "balance method." In this method, the amount of calcium going into the system (the amount consumed) is compared to the amount going out of the system (the amount excreted in urine and feces). The difference between intake and output is called "the balance" and can have a value that is negative, positive, or zero. If you have a positive balance, that means you are retaining more calcium than you are losing. Since 99% of the body's calcium resides in the skeleton, calcium retained during a positive balance reflects an increase in bone mass.

By varying the amount of CCM the girls consumed to produce a wide range of calcium intakes, the Purdue team was able to determine that the maximum average retention of calcium in adolescent girls was 473 mg per day. To put this another way, 473 mg per day is the greatest amount of calcium that can be added to the skeleton during the adolescent years. Of course, since this amount of calcium was the average value, that meant some girls were able to retain more calcium while others retained less. The difference in retention abilities probably reflects genetic factors, which eventually lead to different bone densities as adults. Importantly, the maximum values presented here only represent the highest potential for retaining calcium during adolescence. Whether or not potential is reached depends on calcium intake.

By studying the responses to varied amounts of calcium consumed as CCM, the researchers at Purdue were able to calculate how close the girls were to achieving maximum calcium retention. Currently, the average calcium intake of teenage girls in the United States is just slightly less than 800 mg per day. At this level, the typical girl only achieves 32% of the maximum calcium retention possible. In fact, even in girls who are very efficient at retaining calcium, 800 mg of calcium will only produce about 50% of the maximum retention. The current intake recommendation from the National Academy of Sciences for teenage girls—1,300 mg of calcium per day—is high enough to maximize calcium retention in girls who have exceptionally good abilities to retain calcium. However, for the typical girl, 1,300 mg of calcium will only bring her up to 63%

of her highest possible retention. As calcium intake rises above this level, there is continued improvement in retention. At 2,000 mg, the typical teenage girl will reach about 91% of the maximal calcium retention in her skeleton.

Bone Mass and Fractures in Children

The role of bone building during childhood and adolescence is usually thought of in terms of laying the foundation for a healthy skeleton that we can carry into adulthood. More specifically, maximizing your peak bone mass, which happens mainly before you turn 20 years of age, is a way to reduce your risk of developing osteoporotic fractures during your older years. In fact, many health authorities believe that optimizing peak bone mass is the most important factor for reducing fractures later in life. However, can children reap an immediate benefit of fracture reduction by increasing their bone density by optimizing calcium intake?

Most of researchers' efforts to study the type and number of fractures that occur in our society have focused on adults, particularly older adults, for whom fracture frequency is the greatest. However, we all know that children suffer from fractures, too. As such, quantifying the type and number of these fractures is a job that several research teams around the world have tackled. According to Velimir Matkovic, M.D., Ph.D., director of the Bone and Mineral Metabolism Laboratory at Ohio State University, a group of researchers from the United Kingdom were the first to point out that fractures have a "bimodal," or two-phased, type pattern in the population.[37,38] Obviously, because of osteoporosis, one of the peak phases for fracture occurs during older age. However, the other peak time for fractures is during childhood. Similar observations have been made for children living in the United States, Sweden, and Canada.[39–41] The peak in fractures occurs during puberty, with the most common types of fractures involving the hand and the wrist.

Some of the behaviors that teenagers adopt certainly have a bearing on the increase in fracture frequency. For example, they start driving cars. If you've ever had to pay a car insurance premium for a teenager, you know they are high because these young adults are notorious for having a greater number of accidents. Another important factor is their participation in sports. Although they may have played team or individual sports at an earlier age, the level and intensity of competition increases in the teenage years. In a similar vein, their recreational and playtime activities, such as skating, skiing, biking, and so on, become more daring and more likely to lead to accidents and fractures. However, it's more than just behavior that drives the fracture rates up during adolescence. A number of researchers have reported that a large percentage of the fractures in children, perhaps 30% to 40% of the total, cannot be accounted for by a specific event involving physical activity or motor vehicle accidents.[40] Furthermore, for most of the fractures that can be linked to a specific event, the level of trauma, or force of the event, is considered to be only slight. This has led some in the medical community to suggest that many of these fractures in childhood are misclassified as traumatic and should instead be considered bone fragility fractures, similar to osteoporosis-related fractures.

There is a plausible physical reason to believe that bone fragility is, in fact, the cause of these fractures and that greater bone density will protect kids during this peak fracture phase just as it does in adults. If you look at the age when the fracture rates reach their peak in children, you'll find it occurs at the very same time they are making their greatest gains in height.[41] This is at about age 12 for girls and age 14 for boys. Children can't get taller unless their skeletons get bigger. During this rapid phase of growth, the lengthening and widening of the skeleton (bone size) is outpacing the ability of the body to mineralize the bone. Thus, on a temporary basis, there is a relative reduction in bone density. Since bone density is directly related to bone strength, a weakening of the skeleton occurs during the rapid growth of puberty. In fact, a comparison of children with fractures to those who remain fracture-free shows that average bone density is lower in the fracture group. Thus, maximizing bone density gain during a child's growth and development, including optimizing their calcium intake, will have immediate as well as long-term benefits for fracture reduction.

CHAPTER FIVE

CCM and Bone Building in Adults

- Medical Community Kills Calcium in the 1980s
- CCM and the Rebirth of Calcium in the 1990s
- CCM Prevents Bone Loss
- Building on the Effect of CCM with Other Nutrients
- CCM and Fracture Protection in Men and Women
- Weight Loss, Bone Loss, and CCM

Since 1990, research with CCM has provided a steady stream of landmark discoveries in the area of reducing and preventing bone loss and building bone density in postmenopausal women. Studies with CCM were the first to show there was a difference in the effectiveness of various calcium supplements and that supplementation could significantly reduce bone loss in the spine and hip.[1] This led to additional experiments showing how to build on and increase the effectiveness of CCM by combining it with other nutrients.[2–5] Further work with CCM provided the world's only study showing that bone fractures in both older women and men could be significantly reduced via supplementation.[6] These studies with CCM have not only been on the leading edge but, in many ways, have *defined* the leading edge of the nutrition and bone health movement.

Bone loss is often regarded as a "normal" part of the aging process. I strongly urge you to challenge this concept. . . . Sure, you'd be in better shape now if you had been optimizing nutrition for maximum skeletal health your whole life. But it's not too late.

Bone loss is often regarded as a "normal" part of the aging process. I strongly urge you to challenge this concept. The research is on your side and shows that you can make changes leading to better bone health. Sure, you'd be in better shape now if you had been optimizing nutrition for maximum skeletal health your whole life. But it's not too late. Most people make it to at least age 50 with a skeleton that is strong enough to withstand osteoporotic fractures. In fact, the incidence of fracture is quite low up to this point. However, after age 50, you enter a time of life when fracture risk begins to rise at an increasingly steeper rate.

The lion's share of medical research on the benefits of calcium has clearly been directed at studying its effect on bone loss in postmenopausal women. A lot of water has passed under this bridge. Over the past 10 to 15 years, we've gone from being mired in a controversial, seemingly utter state of confusion about calcium to what approaches being a true consensus in at least one area of nutrition. Some of the most successful results have been generated using CCM supplements. This chapter presents these discoveries and gives you additional information on understanding the role of calcium and other nutrients in bone health.

Medical Community Kills Calcium in the 1980s

With all the news we hear these days about the importance of calcium intake for reducing bone loss in postmenopausal women, it seems strange to look back at a time, not so long ago, when there was little or no agreement about the effectiveness of calcium. In fact, what agreement there was, tipped toward the viewpoint that calcium supplementation was not effective in reducing bone loss in postmenopausal women. In the late 1980s, physicians had little regard for the potential benefit of increased calcium intake. Even more bizarre, this general belief came on the heels of a consensus report from the National Institutes of Health in 1984, recommending calcium intakes of 1,000 to 1,500 mg per day to reduce bone loss. However, when Surgeon General C. Everett Koop, M.D., released his report on Nutrition and Health in 1988, he was unwilling to make a recommendation regarding the benefit of increased calcium intake for reducing age-related bone loss in postmenopausal women.[7]

What happened in the 1980s to cause a downturn in people's interest in calcium? A number of factors were responsible and since hindsight is often 20/20, there is no use in assigning blame to any particular person or group. It is, however, helpful to understand the environment that existed in the late '80s so we can learn from the experience. First, osteoporosis was clearly recognized as an important public health problem. However, the future magnitude of its importance was not fully realized in the context of the increasing average age of the population (the so-called "graying of America"). Fewer researchers and clinicians took a keen interest in the causes and treatments for osteoporosis, compared with the receptive research climate that exists today. Bone densitometers were not in common use. They were used as research tools but were not standard equipment in hospital radiology departments as they are now in many cities.

Second, the overall interest by physicians and consumers in preventative medicine was not nearly as widespread as it is today. Aging baby boomers are seeing the effects of chronic diseases on their parents and are starting to notice the early signs of these diseases in themselves. The boomer generation is turning out to be less willing to take a passive role in their own health and well-being. They are more interested in self-help, prevention, and the prospects of a long, active, and healthy post-retirement life. Physicians are responding to this change in attitude as well. Osteoporosis, like other chronic diseases, used to be thought of in terms of "you either have it or you don't," and we'll wait until you have it to do something. Now, chronic diseases are seen more as a continuum of risk factors. The traumatic event, such as a fracture, a coronary event, the need for insulin, and so on, is not viewed as defining the disease but as an advanced stage of the disease or health condition.

The third factor involved the publication of three scientific research papers in top-tier medical journals, which would be widely and repeatedly cited as evidence against calcium supplementation. The first of these studies appeared in the *British Medical Journal* in 1984.[8] It involved 103 women living in Denmark who were within an average of less than two years since their menopause. These participants were put into one of three groups, depending on their usual dietary calcium intake. The "low" intake group averaged 430 mg of calcium per day, the "medium" group 880 mg per day, and the "high" group 1,640 mg per day. All of the women continued with their normal diets and received an additional 500 mg of calcium per day as a calcium carbonate supplement. Changes in bone mass of the forearm were measured over a two-year period to evaluate the effectiveness of calcium. After two years, there were no significant differences among the three groups; they all lost about 4% of their bone mass.

In early January of 1987, a paper appeared in the *Annals of Internal Medicine* that detailed the effects on bone loss of 1,000 mg of supplemental calcium given as calcium carbonate to postmenopausal women who were within an average of two years since their menopause.[9] A total of 55 women participated in the study for two years. No benefit at all from the calcium was seen in the spine: Loss of bone mass was documented to be 10.5% in the group taking the calcium carbonate supplement and only 9% in the group without supplementation. Bone density in the radius of the arm showed a slight benefit from calcium, with the unsupplemented group losing about 2% and the calcium carbonate group losing 1% of their bone mass.

The final nail in the calcium coffin came approximately two weeks later with a study published in the *New England Journal of Medicine,* the country's most prestigious medical journal.[10] The two previous studies, although supportive of the calcium nay-sayers, had lacked complete scientific rigor in that they were not double-blind, placebo-controlled, or randomized. However, this new study had all the hallmarks of being a well-controlled clinical trial to test the effects of calcium supplementation on bone loss. Twenty-five women within an average of less than two years since their menopause were randomly assigned to either a placebo or 2,000 mg of extra calcium per day supplied as calcium carbonate. Over the two years of the study, changes in bone mass were measured in the forearm, the total body, and the spine. Bone loss was significant in both the calcium carbonate and placebo groups, averaging from 4% to 8%. There was no significant difference between calcium carbonate and placebo treatment for bone loss in the spine and total body. Although the forearm did show some benefit, both groups still had significant bone loss at this site.

CCM and the Rebirth of Calcium in the 1990s

What was wrong with the previous studies of calcium supplementation? Why did they fail to show a benefit? The problem is more a matter of how the studies were interpreted rather than in any particular design flaw. It would finally take a study conducted with CCM to jump-start a renewed interest in the benefits of calcium for reducing bone loss in postmenopausal women.

To begin with, the number of subjects used in these previous studies was relatively small. Bone loss in postmenopausal women is a slow and gradual process with yearly percentage losses in the single digits or even less than 1% in some cases. Of course, these small yearly decreases add up to large decrements in bone mass over time. Consider that a loss of just 1% to 2% per year starting at age 50 means that 20% to 40% of the skeleton is gone by age 70. However, long-term studies of bone loss are expensive to conduct and, in general, it is financially impractical for these studies to go beyond two or three years in length. Thus, fairly large groups of women are needed to detect the small differences in bone loss.

One of the most significant problems in the interpretation of these studies was that they involved women who were very close to menopause. However, the results were extrapolated by the medical community at large and by consumers to include all postmenopausal women regardless of age or years since menopause. Although this was never the intent of the researchers, it happened nonetheless. The researchers, to their credit, did the logical thing by studying women soon after menopause. Bone loss is known to be more rapid right after menopause and then slows to a more gradual rate later. Given the difficulty in studying the small changes in bone that occur with aging, it made sense to focus on the phase of life when bone loss was more rapid and thus could be more easily studied. We now understand that this rapid phase of bone loss during the immediate postmenopausal period is driven primarily by the removal of estrogen from a woman's system—"estrogen deficiency," if you will. Since bone loss during the early postmenopausal period is caused by estrogen deficiency, not calcium deficiency, it can not be corrected by calcium supplementation. Over time, during the first two to five years after menopause, the effect of estrogen withdrawal on bone loss diminishes and the underlying calcium inadequacy common to many postmenopausal women becomes a more important cause of bone loss.[11,12]

A final problem with interpreting the earlier studies of calcium and bone loss in postmenopausal women involves the type of calcium used. All three influential studies discussed earlier used calcium carbonate as the source of supplemental calcium. The failure of calcium carbonate to provide clear-cut benefits for reducing bone loss were extrapolated to mean that no calcium source would be beneficial. This belief was reinforced by yet another study published in the *New England Journal of Medicine* in 1987 that dealt with calcium absorption from different supplemental sources of calcium. A team of researchers from Baylor University measured calcium absorption from milk, calcium carbonate, and a variety of other calcium supplements, including calcium citrate, calcium lactate, and calcium gluconate.[13] They found no significant differences among any of the sources. *However, subsequent studies in both adults and children would show that calcium absorption from CCM was significantly greater than from either milk or calcium carbonate.*[14–19]

CCM Prevents Bone Loss

All of the previous notions surrounding the lack of effectiveness of calcium supplementation to curb bone loss in postmenopausal women were challenged by the first long-term bone study with CCM.[1] The study was primarily funded by the U.S. Department of Agriculture and was conducted at the

Human Nutrition Research Center on Aging at Tufts University. To this day, it remains a unique experiment in the field of calcium nutrition. Published in the *New England Journal of Medicine* in 1990, this study is one of the largest, if not *the* largest, controlled trial of calcium supplementation ever conducted in postmenopausal women. It was the first study to show that, over a two-year period, a calcium supplement could significantly reduce, and in some cases eliminate, bone loss in the spine and hip. Moreover, it was, and is, *the only study to show that calcium supplements differ in their effectiveness on bone.*

Three hundred and one healthy postmenopausal women from the Boston, Massachusetts, area were recruited to participate. They were randomly assigned in a double-blind fashion to either a placebo, 500 mg of supplemental calcium per day in the form of calcium carbonate, or 500 mg of supplemental calcium per day in the form of CCM. For two years, the women maintained their normal diets and were instructed to take their supplement (placebo, calcium carbonate, or CCM) at bedtime. Bone density was measured in the spine, hip, and forearm.

An important design element built into the study was to evaluate the response to calcium supplementation as a function of years since menopause. Thus, the women were grouped according to whether their menopause was within five years or less from the start of the study ("early postmenopausal women") or whether it had been more than five years since their menopause ("late postmenopausal women"). As the other researchers had seen in their previous studies, the early postmenopausal women lost bone, particularly in the spine, and there was no significant effect from calcium supplementation. This was an important observation to make because it anchored the present study with CCM to the previous studies of calcium supplementation and thus laid the foundation for new discoveries to be accepted.

In the group of late postmenopausal women, calcium supplementation, particularly in the form of CCM, had a dramatic effect on bone loss. At all three skeletal sites (spine, hip, and forearm), the group of women taking CCM differed significantly from the placebo group and had no statistically significant loss of bone. In contrast, the calcium carbonate group gave an intermediate response that did not significantly differ from the placebo at any of the three bone sites. Average bone loss in the spine during the two years of the study was about 2% in both the placebo and calcium carbonate groups. However, CCM reduced bone loss in the spine by about 60%, bringing it down to less than 1%. At the hip and forearm, the percentage of change in bone density in the group receiving CCM was a positive number, averaging +0.4% to +1.0%, whereas the placebo group lost about 1%. Figure 5-1 illustrates the net difference in bone density between the women taking CCM and those taking a typical calcium supplement or a placebo.

Building on the Effect of CCM with Other Nutrients

The study of CCM and postmenopausal women published in the *New England Journal of Medicine* was truly a landmark in the field of calcium supplementation and bone loss. It showed for the first time that calcium supplementation (with CCM) could have a major impact on bone loss in the spine, hip, and forearm. It also showed that supplementation with CCM was more effective than using calcium carbonate. However, despite the very positive results of this study, there was still room for improvement. Let me explain. Bone loss had been clearly halted during a two-year period at the hip and forearm. However, the

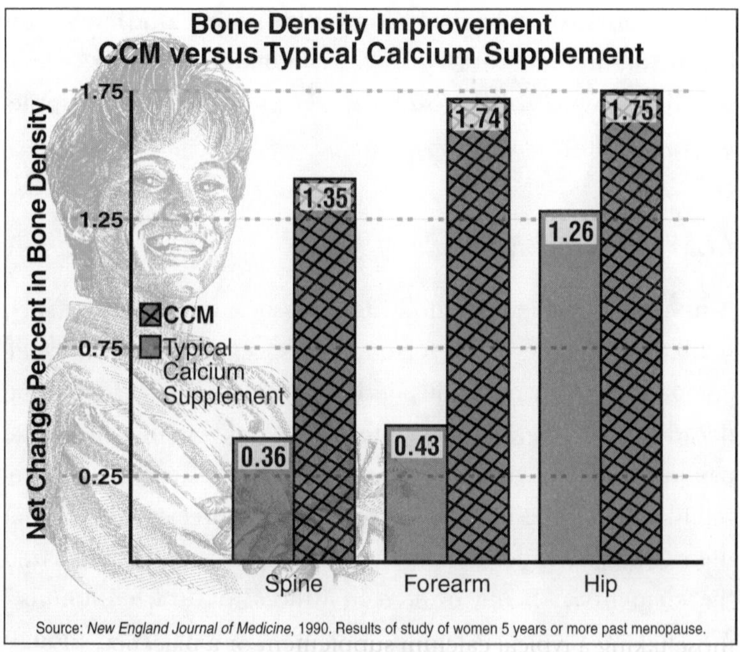

Figure 5-1

CCM reduced bone loss significantly, which translates to a positive net gain or percent improvement in bone density.

spine was proving to be a problem site for nutritional intervention. Although CCM had significantly reduced bone loss in the spine by 60%, the average change in bone density was still tending toward the negative side. The concept that the spine was less responsive than other bone sites to calcium therapy was also propounded by a researcher named Robert Graham Cumming from the University of Sydney, Australia. He compiled a review of the world's literature on the effect of calcium intake on bone mass and found that it was common for supplemental calcium to have some positive effect in the forearm but not in the spine.[20] As such, we became interested in exploring the possibility that the positive effect of CCM in the spine could be improved by combining it with other nutrients. This led to additional work with postmenopausal women, which would produce further novel discoveries in the area of supplementation and bone loss.

CCM Plus Trace Minerals

A number of minerals found in our tissues are present in such small amounts they are referred to as trace minerals or trace elements. The concentrations of these minerals are so small that, decades ago, researchers doing early work on the elemental composition of living things could not measure them accurately. Therefore, instead of reporting a precise value from their analytical experiments, the researchers simply categorized the elements as being present in "traces" or "trace amounts." This moniker, "trace mineral," is still used today even though our analytical methodologies have improved to the point where the trace minerals can be accurately measured.

The trace minerals or elements that are currently recognized as essential for human health include iron, zinc, iodine, selenium, copper, manganese, chromium, and molybdenum.[21] Fluoride doesn't really meet the criteria for being an essential element. However, because of its positive effects on dental health, fluoride is usually included as belonging to the group of essential trace elements.

A number of other trace elements have been demonstrated to be essential for the health of certain animals, but the data are not strong enough to provide any estimate for a safe and adequate intake recommendation in humans. This group is comprised of boron, silicon, nickel, and arsenic. Further down the list of possible essential trace elements are vanadium, tin, lithium, lead, and cadmium. For these trace elements (sometimes called "ultratrace elements"), there has been some evidence of deficiency produced in laboratory animals. To produce a deficiency, the animals need to be kept in special environments designed to prevent exposure to even the tiniest amount of the elements. No benefits to humans are known at this time, and if we require any of these trace elements, it is very likely that our need is extremely small and easily met via environmental exposure.[21]

Bone turnover . . . involves both the breakdown (bone resorption) and building (bone formation) of bone tissue. . . . Bone loss during aging represents an imbalance during the remodeling process, in which more bone tissue is removed than synthesized.

The essential function of several trace minerals for normal bone metabolism has been recognized for about four decades.[22] The trace elements needed for bone health are in the group of trace minerals known to be required by humans. They serve specific metabolic roles that are key to the normal functioning of the bone turnover process. Bone turnover is an important concept to grasp for understanding how bones work and how to keep the skeleton healthy. Bone turnover occurs throughout the skeleton at all ages. It involves both the breakdown (bone resorption) and building (bone formation) of bone tissue by specific bone cells called osteoblasts and osteoclasts. Bone loss during aging represents an imbalance during the remodeling process, in which more bone tissue is removed than is synthesized. Bone is composed of two basic materials, a protein component and a mineral component. During the resorption and formation process, both the protein and mineral components are removed and then added back. However, the timing of these events is such that the protein component of bone is synthesized first and then, and only then, the protein component becomes mineralized. A defect in the control or functioning of either the protein synthesis or the mineralization process is ultimately the cause of bone loss.

The trace minerals zinc, copper, and manganese are intimately involved in synthesizing the protein component of bone, whereas calcium is used during the mineralization of bone. Deficiency of each of these trace minerals has been shown to have adverse effects on bone metabolism in animals. Zinc is required for protein metabolism within all cells because it is essential in the regulation of DNA and RNA, the genetic blueprints from which all proteins are made. Copper is needed by an enzyme (lysyl oxidase) responsible for the proper formation of the proteins collagen and elastin, the main proteins within bone. Manganese is required by enzymes called glycosyltransferases. These enzymes make specialized proteins in bone that are present in small amounts but that help regulate the bone turnover and mineralization processes.

Despite the documented involvement of these trace minerals in bone metabolism over the past 40 years, no one had ever performed a study to measure their effects on bone loss in postmenopausal women. In fact, the first and only study to date to investigate the potential benefit of trace mineral supplementation was a collaborative effort between the University of California at San Diego (UCSD) and the Procter & Gamble Company.[3] The study, funded by the National Institutes of Health and Procter & Gamble, was conducted with participants living around the UCSD campus in La Jolla, California.

Fifty-nine postmenopausal women, with an average age of 66 years, completed a trial of the effect of CCM plus trace mineral supplementation on bone loss. To participate, the women had to be in good general health and not be taking any supplements or drugs known to impact bone metabolism. The study was double-blind, placebo-controlled, and randomized. Women were assigned to one of four supplement groups. One group was given a placebo, another group received trace minerals, another group received CCM, and the final group got both CCM and trace minerals.

The women continued with their normal diets and activities throughout the study. The groups taking CCM received an extra 1,000 mg of calcium per day. The groups taking trace minerals received an extra 15 mg of zinc, 5 mg of manganese, and 2.5 mg of copper per day. These amounts of supplemental zinc, manganese, and copper are very close to the current intake recommendations. The Recommended Dietary Allowance (RDA) for zinc set by the National Academy of Sciences (NAS) is 12 mg. The estimated safe and adequate daily intake set by the NAS is 2–5 mg for manganese and 1.5–3.0 mg for copper.[21]

Assessment of the participants' diets showed an average daily calcium consumption from dietary sources of about 600 mg per day. This value closely agrees with national statistics for calcium intake by postmenopausal women of this age group.[23] The intake of zinc, copper, and manganese from the diet was not measured. However, from other studies, we know that intakes of all three trace minerals typically fall below recommended amounts. For example, a recent national survey conducted by the U.S. Department of Agriculture found that 85% of postmenopausal women consume less than 100% of the RDA for zinc.[23] An extensive dietary analysis by the FDA (Food and Drug Administration) found that the average copper intake by adult females was only 0.9 mg per day. This value is 40% below the lowest range of intake estimated to be safe and adequate by the National Academy of Sciences. The same study showed that typical manganese intakes were 2.2 mg per day in adult women, compared to the safe and adequate range of 2–5 mg.[24]

CCM completely halted bone loss in the hip and forearm and reduced bone loss in the spine by 60%.

Changes in bone density in the spine were measured during the two-year period the women took the supplements or the placebo. The spine was a fortuitous bone site to focus on, based on the findings from the previous study of CCM in postmenopausal women. Recall that the previous controlled trial with CCM was the first study to show that a calcium source could benefit the spine, hip, and forearm. CCM completely halted bone loss in the hip and forearm and reduced bone loss in the spine by 60%. Calcium carbonate supplements had no significant effect on bone loss in the spine. Thus, the spine was shown to be more resistant than other skeletal sites to calcium nutritional therapy.

In the study of CCM and trace minerals, loss of bone density in the spine was greatest in the placebo group (–3.5%). The effect of trace minerals alone (zinc, copper, and manganese) reduced bone loss by 45%, but this was not statistically different from the placebo. The overall effect of CCM supplementation was significant and spinal bone loss was reduced by 65%. This value was very close to what was found in the previous study for CCM's effect on the spine. *In the group of women receiving CCM plus trace minerals, spinal bone density loss was completely halted.* The average change in bone density for this group was +1.5% compared to the placebo group's loss of –3.5%, a net difference of 5%.

This study reveals new and potentially important facts regarding nutritional approaches for reducing bone loss in postmenopausal women. It shows that more comprehensive strategies are needed, which involve support of both the mineralization and protein-synthesis processes in bone. A report of our findings was published in 1994 in the *Journal of Nutrition,* the official journal of the American Society of Nutritional Sciences.[3] Subsequently, a number of research groups around the country have become interested in the role of trace minerals in postmenopausal bone loss and are actively working to generate more information.

CCM Plus Vitamin D

Another way to try and build on the effectiveness of CCM for reducing bone loss in postmenopausal women is to combine it with vitamin D. Vitamin D has long been known to be intimately linked to calcium and bone metabolism. Technically, vitamin D is not really a vitamin at all. It's a hormone our own bodies can make via exposure to sunshine. That's why vitamin D is known as the "sunshine vitamin." Our skin contains a precursor of vitamin D ("provitamin D"). The ultraviolet light in sunshine triggers a reaction that leads to the rapid conversion of provitamin D into vitamin D. However, with aging, we become much less efficient at vitamin D synthesis. Our skin becomes thinner with age and the amount of provitamin D stored within the skin goes down drastically. Studies with healthy young people (younger than age 31) and older people (older than age 61) show that older people can produce only one-fourth the amount of vitamin D from the same amount of ultraviolet exposure.[25]

Another important factor affecting your ability to synthesize vitamin D is the season of the year and where you live. We all know that winter is characterized by "short days" (less sunlight). However, it's not only the amount of sunlight that changes with the season but the intensity of the sunlight's ultraviolet radiation. During the winter, in points north of Atlanta, Georgia, the intensity of ultraviolet radiation is not strong enough to trigger the vitamin D–synthesizing pathway. The farther north you go, the less intense the ultraviolet rays become and the fewer months out of the year you have to make vitamin D from sunshine. Michael Holick, M.D., has done pioneering work on the effect of latitude, season, and time of day on vitamin D synthesis from sunshine. Dr. Holick is the director of the

Vitamin D, Skin, and Bone Research Lab and Chief of Endocrinology at Boston University's Medical Center. According to his studies, from November through February, people living in Boston, Massachusetts, can't make any vitamin D from sunshine. As he likes to put it for emphasis, "You can lay outside naked all day and it won't do you any good." In contrast, people living in Los Angeles can make vitamin D all year long. But remember, even if you live in a more southerly latitude, your ability to make vitamin D from sunshine greatly diminishes with age. That's why greater vitamin D intake, including the use of supplements, is often recommended for people beginning at age 50.

Midday sunshine has the most intense ultraviolet radiation and is therefore most capable of promoting vitamin D synthesis. Of course, midday sun is also the most dangerous for increasing your risk of getting skin cancer and wrinkles. Related to this, sunscreen preparations that effectively protect the skin also block vitamin D synthesis. In addition, sunshine that passes through windows is ineffective for promoting vitamin D.[25]

It may seem difficult to balance our need for adequate sunlight exposure (which is also one of life's simple pleasures) to the potential risks. However, as Dr. Holick points out, there is a way to intelligently use sunshine. First, it doesn't take very much exposure to get the vitamin D synthesis job done (assuming you live far enough south and it's the right time of year). Exposing your hands, arms, and face two to three times a week for a few minutes will do it. There is no need to get sunburned! In fact, Dr Holick recommends that the time you are exposed should be about one-half the time it takes for even a slight sunburn to occur. Second, kids and young adults generally don't need to worry about vitamin D. They're more efficient at making vitamin D, more apt to spend time outside, and less likely to carefully and completely apply sunscreen. Even at the higher latitudes, younger people can make and store enough vitamin D to have adequate levels during the winter months. Third, older individuals should regularly consume at least 400 IU of vitamin D per day from dietary or supplemental sources. The current recommended intake for vitamin D is 400 IU for people ages 51 to 70 years old and 600 IU for those past 70.[26]

In concert with the theme of older individuals requiring supplemental vitamin D, especially if they live in more northern latitudes, a study was conducted in postmenopausal women living in the Boston, Massachusetts, area. The study tested the benefit of adding 400 IU of vitamin D per day on top of CCM supplementation. This study was primarily funded by the U.S. Department of Agriculture and was conducted at the Human Nutrition Research Center on Aging at Tufts University.[2]

Subjects in the study were 249 healthy postmenopausal women with an average age of 61 years. The study was randomized, double-blind, and placebo-controlled. All the women received a calcium supplement containing CCM, which brought their total calcium intake (diet plus supplement) up to an average of 800 mg per day. In addition to the calcium supplement, one-half of the women received a supplement containing 400 IU of vitamin D; the other women took a placebo. The intake of vitamin D from dietary sources averaged 100 IU per day, which is typical of intakes by postmenopausal women. Thus, with supplementation, the group receiving extra vitamin D received a total (diet plus supplement) of 500 IU per day. (Note: At the time this study was conducted, the RDAs for calcium and vitamin D in postmenopausal women were 800 mg and 200 IU, respectively. The intake recommendations have subsequently been increased to

1,200 mg of calcium and 400 IU of vitamin D by the National Academy of Sciences.)

A unique aspect of the study was the way bone mass measurements were taken. Bone density was assessed three times during a 12-month period in order to measure changes occurring in the wintertime, summertime, and over the entire year. Before this study was conducted, other researchers had speculated that bone loss might be more severe during the winter months because of inadequate sunshine and vitamin D synthesis. However, this was the first study to actually measure changes in bone density as a function of the season of the year. The results of the study were remarkable, in that they showed an amplitude to changes in bone density. Like a pendulum swinging back and forth, bone density went up in the summer and down in the winter.

In the group of women receiving the supplement with CCM only (no vitamin D), the up and down swings were equal so that no bone density was lost over the entire 12-month period. This result agreed with the other studies of CCM supplementation in postmenopausal women, showing that it has a major positive impact on halting bone loss. *However, an exciting new discovery was that the addition of the vitamin D supplement along with CCM resulted in a significant gain in bone density in the spine of about 1%.* The increase in spinal bone density was due to a reduction in the wintertime loss of bone. Considered together with the study using CCM plus trace mineral supplementation, this study of CCM plus vitamin D shows that there are two separate ways to build on and improve the effectiveness of CCM for stopping bone loss in the spine. It is interesting to speculate on what the effects would be of taking the complete triad: CCM, trace minerals, and vitamin D. Although this combination has yet to be tested, common sense would say it represents a more comprehensive nutritional approach with greater overall benefits.

At this point, you are probably wondering how to get adequate amounts of vitamin D and trace minerals into your diet. The main food source of vitamin D is fluid milk, because it has vitamin D added. However, to obtain 400 IU of vitamin D you need to drink a quart of milk per day. Furthermore, although milk is a good reliable source of calcium, a study published in the *New England Journal of Medicine* showed that the amount of vitamin D listed on the label and the amount of vitamin D actually in the milk don't always match up.[27,28] Of the milk samples analyzed, 14% had no vitamin D, and one-half of the samples had less than 80% of the amount claimed on the label. Also, because milk is fortified with vitamin D (or is supposed to be), many people mistakenly believe that other dairy products are fortified, too. They're not—neither yogurt nor cheese, only milk. Once you get past milk, the list of viable choices for adding vitamin D to your daily diet without supplementation becomes very short. Liver, egg yolks, fatty fish, and cod liver oil are the richest natural sources.

With respect to the trace minerals, animal products are the highest sources for zinc and copper. Meat—especially red meat—oysters, fish, and egg yolks are high in zinc. Copper is present in the highest amounts in seafood, nuts, and seeds, and if you have copper piping in your home, you may get significant quantities from tap water. Most of our dietary manganese comes from whole grains and cereals. Animal products, dairy, meat, fish, and so on, are poor sources of manganese. Usually, one-a-day type multivitamin-multimineral supplements have 100% of the RDA of zinc, copper, and manganese. But check the label to be sure.

CCM and Fracture Protection in Men and Women

A hierarchy of effectiveness exists for products containing calcium. This hierarchy contains four levels:

1. Calcium content
2. Calcium absorption
3. Bone density benefits
4. Fracture protection

Obviously, if a product contains no calcium, there can be no calcium nutritional benefit. However, due to differences in the bioavailability of calcium, the presence of calcium, per se, says very little about the effectiveness of the product. As detailed in Chapter 2 on calcium absorption, we know that bioavailability, or degree of absorption, has a tenfold range, depending on the calcium source. This means that two products containing the same amount of calcium can vary widely in terms of the amount of calcium actually delivered to your bloodstream and ultimately to your skeleton.

This brings us to the second level of benefit in the calcium hierarchy, calcium absorption. In addition to the amount of calcium that is contained in a food or supplement, the extent of nutritional benefit is linked to how well the calcium is absorbed. The vast majority of calcium-containing products has not been measured for calcium absorption. In contrast, the research completed on CCM has shown that it resides in the upper range of the calcium absorption spectrum, providing significantly greater calcium absorption than both milk and calcium carbonate.

The third level of effectiveness in the calcium hierarchy involves bone mass benefits. While calcium absorption is certainly an important attribute for defining the potential benefit of a calcium product, absorption tests are typically very short-term in nature. Usually, calcium absorption is measured from a single dose or meal. On the other hand, changes in bone density are necessarily made over a fairly long time period and directly address the impact of calcium on the skeleton. For example, the studies showing CCM's benefit to bone density in children and postmenopausal women were six months to four years in duration. Bone density is highly predictive of bone strength. As such, it's not surprising that fracture risk is significantly correlated to bone density. Thus, a calcium product with clinically documented benefits to bone density is more certain to deliver fracture protection than a product that has only been shown to deliver absorbable calcium.

In principle, lower levels in the calcium benefit hierarchy lead to higher and higher benefits and ultimately to fracture protection (the greatest benefit). However, simply hypothesizing that benefits should be present is quite different from actually showing it. Hypothesizing is hoping; seeing is believing. As you move up the benefit hierarchy from any lower level to the next higher level, the benefit of calcium may not prove out. For example, spinach is one of the highest calcium-containing vegetables; however, hardly any of its calcium is absorbable. The calcium from calcium carbonate is known to be absorbed as well as that in milk; however, a study of men given 1,000 mg of extra calcium per day as calcium carbonate plus vitamin D showed no effect on bone loss.[29] Vitamin D is known to be intimately involved in calcium and bone metabolism; however, a large study (2,600 subjects) of older men and women given a placebo or 400 IU of vitamin D for three years showed no significant difference in fracture rates.[30] These examples show that a benefit from the lower levels of the hierarchy does not necessarily translate to a higher level benefit. Thus, to be certain you receive the full spectrum of benefits, you need to choose a calcium source that has shown effectiveness at all levels of the hierarchy.

A number of previous studies with CCM have shown that it clearly delivers benefits from the first three levels in the calcium hierarchy. To test whether CCM could also deliver the fourth and highest level of benefit (fracture protection), a study was conducted with 389 healthy older men and women. This was a three-year, double-blind, randomized study in which subjects received either a placebo or a supplement combination of 500 mg of calcium as CCM and 700 IU of vitamin D. The results were published in the *New England Journal of Medicine* in 1997.[6] All of the subjects were age 65 or older (average age—71 years). This was the world's first study to measure the effects of calcium and vitamin D supplementation on bone loss and fracture incidence in healthy older men and women living at home. These were regular older folks, living on their own and taking care of themselves. They had made it this far with pretty good bone health but were in the phase of life when osteoporotic fractures were a common and ever-increasing threat to their independence.

During the study, bone density was measured in the hip, spine, and total body with state-of-the-art equipment. Peripheral fractures (feet, ankles, legs, hips, pelvis, ribs, hands, arms, shoulders, clavicle, and face) were verified using x-rays and hospital records. Calcium and vitamin D from dietary sources were measured and shown to average about 700–800 mg (calcium) and 200 IU vitamin D per day. There was no significant difference between the groups in their level of physical activity or number of falls.

Bone density changes in the group receiving CCM plus vitamin D were highly significant compared to the placebo group. *Over the three years of supplementation, no loss of bone density occurred in the spine, hip, or total body in the men and women taking CCM with vitamin D. In fact, small but significant increases in bone density occurred at all three sites.* The net changes in bone density (difference between the placebo and CCM plus vitamin D groups) were +1.3% in the hip, spine, and total body.

Osteoporotic fractures were reduced by 64% in the CCM plus vitamin D group compared to the placebo group. Most fractures occurring during the study were osteoporotic in nature (low trauma, fragility fractures). However, even if you included all fractures, the effect was still significant and showed a 54% reduction in the CCM plus vitamin D group.

Weight loss from dieting is a recently identified risk factor that can accelerate bone loss.

Recall that CCM alone, or combined with vitamin D or trace minerals, had been shown in previous studies to be highly beneficial to bone density in postmenopausal women. However, this new study was the first to show a bone density benefit to men and a fracture protection benefit for healthy, older men and women combined. Few studies with men are available to compare these results with, and the only other one that used a combination of calcium and vitamin D was published in 1990.[29] Compared to the recent CCM plus vitamin D study, the men in this earlier study were younger (average age—58 years) and received greater amounts of supplementation: 1,000 mg of calcium as calcium carbonate and 1,000 IU of vitamin D for three years. The men lost bone density in the spine and forearm, and the combination of calcium carbonate and vitamin D had no effect on bone loss. For women, the only other similar study was published in 1992.[31] The women is this study were older (average age—84 years), received greater amounts of supplementation (1,200 mg of calcium as calcium phosphate and 800 IU of vitamin D for 18 months), and had a fracture reduction that was only one-half as effective as CCM plus vitamin D (28% versus 64% with CCM/vitamin D).

Weight Loss, Bone Loss, and CCM

Weight loss from dieting is a recently identified risk factor that can accelerate bone loss. Dieting to lose body weight is quite common in America, due to the high prevalence of obesity in our population. Individuals who are chronically overweight usually cycle through bouts of weight loss and weight gain, so-called "yo-yo" dieting, which may have a cumulative negative effect on the skeleton. One-third of the children in America are clinically obese and efforts to lose weight during the critical bone-building years of childhood and adolescence could reduce their peak bone mass formation and increase their lifetime risk for osteoporosis.

To address this emerging concern, researchers at Rutgers and Columbia Universities conducted a study of the effects of CCM supplementation on bone loss during weight loss in postmenopausal women.[32] Thirty-one women with an average age of 58 years and average body weight of 194 pounds completed the study. For six months, the women participated in a weight-loss program and received either a placebo or a CCM supplement containing 1,000 mg of calcium per day. Both groups of women lost the same amount of weight, an average of 19 pounds. *The weight-loss group receiving CCM showed no bone loss in the total body.* In contrast, bone density decreased significantly in the placebo group, with an average loss of 1.7%.

CHAPTER SIX

Can Too Much Calcium Hurt Me?

- **Kidney Stones**
- **Calcium's Negative Interaction with Other Minerals**
- **Milk-Alkali Syndrome**
- **Calcium Supplements and Lead**

We all know that too much of anything, even a good thing, can be harmful. Calcium is a fairly innocuous mineral, and the upper limit of intake that health authorities usually recommend ranges from 2,000–2,500 mg per day.[1,2] For the most part, this upper range limit reflects the absence of data showing harm below it, rather than the presence of data showing harm above it. There are so few otherwise healthy people consuming calcium above these levels that we don't know how safe it is. Rare reports in the scientific literature of calcium toxicity usually involve some other mitigating circumstance combined with a very high calcium intake. These rare cases are usually classified as a condition called "milk-alkali syndrome," which you can read about later in this chapter. The most recent analysis (1997) of the risk of too much calcium was conducted by the National Academy of Sciences.[2] After reviewing the available information, they set a tolerable upper intake level of 2,500 mg of calcium for individuals ages one year and older. The upper intake level is believed to be the amount above which risk for adverse effects of calcium begin to rise. For adults, this value is considered to be conservative.

The most common concern people have about the safety of calcium involves kidney stones. Thus, I've devoted a fair amount of space in this chapter to putting this risk, or *lack* of risk, into perspective. To give you a quick peek under the tent, the information on this topic actually shows that calcium intake is *protective* against kidney stones.

A major nutritional risk from higher calcium intake that many people are unaware of is that calcium has been shown to interfere with the utilization of other essential minerals.[3,4] However, this is another area of calcium nutrition where calcium sources behave differently. CCM has been well studied and has been found to lack this tendency to interfere with other minerals.[5–9]

Kidney Stones

Kidney stones are crystals that can cause obstruction of urine flow, bleeding, and localized damage to kidney tissue. When urine becomes supersaturated with stone-forming components, the components slowly precipitate and form crystals. It has been estimated that approximately 12% of Americans will have a kidney stone at some point in their lives.[2] It's extremely rare for children or adolescents to form kidney stones. Usually the age at which the first stone occurs is 20 years or older, with the average age being about 40. Men are much more likely to form kidney stones than women. The male to female ratio is about four to one. Stone recurrence is quite common, with an average length of time between stones of 2.5 years.

Calcium Protects Against Kidney Stones

People with kidney stones are frequently counseled by their doctors to reduce dietary calcium intake. The rationale for this advice is more intuitive than empirical in nature. Most kidney stones contain calcium, and decreasing dietary calcium intake will reduce urinary output of calcium. Thus, doctors have mistakenly held on to the notion that reducing calcium intake will protect against kidney stone formation.

Despite the long-standing practice of encouraging low calcium intake, there is no data showing that dietary calcium causes kidney stones. In fact, studies performed to explore this relationship have found that calcium intake is the same in stone-formers and in those without stones. Nevertheless, the belief that stone formation is linked to dietary calcium intake has persisted.

This myth about calcium and kidney stones was debunked by a study funded by the National Institutes of Health and reported in the *New England Journal of Medicine* in 1993.[10] Researchers from Harvard University conducted a four-year study in 45,000 subjects to measure the relationship between dietary calcium intake and the risk of kidney stone formation. The subjects were all men, age 40 years or older, who had no previous history of stones. This was an ideal group to investigate because kidney stones are more common in men than women, and at least one-half of all men have their first kidney stone after age 40.

A diet low in calcium has no benefit and may actually be detrimental. Low calcium intake increases the risk for kidney stones and provides inadequate amounts of calcium for optimal bone health.

The researchers found the exact opposite of what had been believed for so many years. Higher calcium intakes did not increase the risk of kidney stones. In fact, there was a significant *inverse* relationship between calcium intake and kidney stone formation. That is to say, the greater the men's calcium intake, the less likely their chance of developing a kidney stone. The group of men comprising the highest one-fifth of calcium consumers had an average calcium intake of about 1,300 mg per day and a 34% lower risk of kidney stones than the group with the lowest one-fifth of calcium intake (average intake of about 500 mg per day). This study shows that encouraging a diet low in calcium has no benefit and may actually be detrimental.[11] Low calcium intake increases the risk for kidney stones and provides inadequate amounts of calcium for optimal bone health. Similar results were found by the same researchers in a subsequent study of women.[12] That is, kidney stone risk was inversely associated with calcium intake. Risk was reduced by about 35% in highest versus lowest calcium-consuming women. However, in this study, the use of supplemental calcium was associated with a 20% greater risk of stone formation. Importantly, the researchers suggested that the common practice of taking supplemental calcium without a meal may have contributed to the increased stone risk associated with supplementation.

Importance of Oxalate in Kidney Stone Formation

Why is calcium protective against kidney stones? Admittedly, it does seem counter-intuitive. To understand the mechanism for this protective effect, you need to understand more about the composition of kidney stones. Although 85% or more of all kidney stones contain calcium, the calcium that's in the stone must be complexed with another material to form a stone. There's no such thing as a pure calcium kidney stone. The most common complexing material is called oxalate. The calcium-oxalate complex is extremely insoluble and 80% of all stones are mainly composed of calcium-oxalate. The concentration of oxalate in the urine is a more important cause of calcium oxalate formation than calcium itself is. Small increases in urine oxalate concentration can easily tip the balance in favor of calcium-oxalate precipitation, whereas larger increases in calcium concentration are needed for the same relative effect.

Oxalate is found in foods of vegetable origin. Some of the higher sources include spinach, chives, rhubarb, tea, parsley, radish, collards, carrots, brussels sprouts, garlic, nuts, sweet potatoes, and chocolate.[13] You absorb oxalate from your food and excrete it in urine. As I mentioned previously, calcium-oxalate is extremely insoluble. That's why it is the most likely candidate material for forming kidney stones. However, the same insolubility property can work in your favor to reduce the oxalate absorption from food. This is what the Harvard researchers hypothesized to explain their findings for the protective effect of calcium intake on kidney stone formation. They suggested that calcium from the diet could combine with oxalate from the diet to form calcium-oxalate in the intestine. The calcium-oxalate would precipitate in the gut and not be absorbed.[10]

CCM Reduces Oxalate Absorption

A fair amount of indirect proof exists for the role of calcium in reducing oxalate absorption and, therefore, oxalate excretion in urine. For example, several studies have shown that reducing calcium intake in either kidney stone patients or normal subjects is associated with an increase in urine oxalate excretion. A subgroup of the population that forms stones has a condition called hypercalciuria, which means they excrete abnormally high amounts of calcium in the urine. Even in these individuals, the restriction of dietary calcium intake has been shown to increase the risk for stone formation by favoring a higher urinary output of oxalate.

Although numerous studies had shown an inverse relationship between calcium intake and oxalate excretion, direct evidence of the ability of calcium to block oxalate absorption was lacking until a study involving CCM was published in 1997.[14] Researchers at the University of Wyoming were able to directly follow a dose of oxalate given to both normal and stone-forming persons. They fed them an amount of oxalate that was equivalent to a high oxalate-containing meal. The oxalate dose was given three times, once with no calcium and twice with 300 mg of calcium supplied as calcium carbonate or CCM. The key factor in this experiment, which allowed the researchers to draw firm conclusions, was the use of a special type of oxalate made by the Cambridge Isotope Laboratory in Massachusetts. This special form of oxalate contained a stable (nonradioactive) isotope of carbon (carbon forms the backbone of the oxalate molecule). This allowed the researchers to specifically tell if the oxalate they fed their subjects was absorbed and excreted in the urine.

Calcium had a significant effect on blocking oxalate absorption and excretion in both the kidney stone–forming subjects and the control group. Compared to the oxalate test when no calcium was given, oxalate excretion from the oral dose was reduced 56% by calcium carbonate and 60% by CCM. Importantly, although part of the calcium dose was tied up by oxalate to prevent its absorption, the researchers reported that CCM was still able to provide significantly greater calcium bioavailability than calcium carbonate.

Some final notes on kidney stone risk. One way to reduce your chances of forming a kidney stone, without regard to calcium or oxalate intake and excretion, is to drink plenty of water—at least eight glasses per day. Increasing your fluid intake will increase your urine volume, causing a dilution of all urinary constituents. Although you still excrete the same total amount of calcium, oxalate, and other urine components, their concentrations will be reduced by the greater volume of urine. The other factor to keep in mind is that CCM is composed of a combination of calcium with two organic acids, citric acid and malic acid. Just as you absorb oxalate (oxalic acid) from your diet, you also absorb citrate (citric acid) and malate (malic acid). The important difference is that the calcium-oxalate complex is extremely insoluble whereas calcium citrate malate is very soluble. For this reason, increasing the citrate and malate concentration in urine will be protective against kidney stones.[15,16] In fact, potassium citrate is sometimes used in the clinical management of kidney stone patients. Thus, CCM has a double potential benefit relative to kidney stone risk—it reduces oxalate absorption and supplies citrate and malate.

Calcium's Negative Interaction with Other Minerals

Calcium is known to negatively interact with other essential minerals.[4] It does so in a way that limits the absorption or utilization of the other minerals. Calcium is not alone in this regard. There are multiple mineral-to-mineral interactions that have been documented in both animal and human studies. However, the recent attention and emphasis being placed on the need to substantially increase our calcium intake in order to achieve optimal bone health has also served to draw attention to the possible adverse effects of calcium. From a nutritional point of view, the potential adverse consequence of primary concern is this interaction between calcium and other minerals.

The negative interaction between calcium and other minerals can work in both directions. That is, other minerals can also limit the utilization of calcium. However, there is normally so much more calcium around than the other minerals that we usually think of the interaction as being unidirectional. For example, the average intakes of zinc, iron, and calcium by postmenopausal women are 9 mg, 13 mg, and 600 mg, respectively.[17]

It does not take excessive amounts of calcium to cause a negative interaction with other minerals. Indeed, as you will see in the following sections, amounts below the recommended levels of intake for optimizing bone health can dramatically depress absorption. However, as you will also see, not all calcium sources behave the same. The studies done with CCM show that it has the ability to deliver highly bioavailable calcium without a negative effect on other minerals.[5–9]

The studies done with CCM show that it has the ability to deliver highly bioavailable calcium without a negative effect on other minerals.

One suggestion that has been made to prevent calcium's interference with other minerals is to take calcium supplements between meals. Although this is sound advice on one level, the suggestion has a double edge. On one hand, since calcium must be consumed together with the other minerals for the negative interaction to occur, taking your supplement separate from meals should prevent the problem. On the other hand, this practice may limit the bioavailability of calcium because it has been shown in healthy adults that consumption of a meal boosts calcium absorption.[18] Furthermore, older people with a reduced ability to produce stomach acid will absorb almost no calcium from calcium carbonate unless they take it with a meal.[19] For more information on this topic, see the section on the importance of calcium solubility and stomach acid in Chapter 2, "Maximize Your Calcium Absorption."

One way out of this box is to use CCM. *It provides high calcium absorption with or without a meal and is quite "friendly" to other minerals in terms of not limiting their absorption.* Another approach would be to take some of your calcium supplement with meals and some without. Taking a divided dose of calcium will give you more absorbable calcium than taking it all at once and will help limit negative interactions with other minerals. If you choose to apply this approach, one of the best times to take part of your supplemental calcium is right before bedtime. This helps keep the body supplied with calcium while you sleep and limits the bone resorption (break down) that normally occurs during the overnight fast. Another thing you can do is to be sure to consume the recommended amounts of the minerals that calcium can interfere with. Also, remember that if you exclusively use foods to meet your calcium needs (either naturally high in calcium or fortified), the same mineral-to-mineral negative interaction applies. Dairy products such as milk and cheese have been shown to be at least as potent as calcium supplements in reducing mineral absorption.[3,6]

Calcium-Iron Interaction

Historically, one of the best known mineral-to-mineral interactions is between calcium and iron. The interaction has been repeatedly studied with a number of calcium sources, and calcium has clearly been shown to reduce iron absorption from a meal.[3] The more calcium is consumed, the greater the inhibitory effect on iron absorption. However, the greatest changes occur with relatively low amounts of calcium, essentially reaching a plateau at 300 mg. Milk and cheese have been shown to reduce iron absorption by about 60% to 65%. Calcium phosphate, hydroxyapatite (a form of calcium phosphate), and calcium carbonate reduce iron absorption by 55% to 60%. Calcium citrate is a bit more forgiving, reducing iron absorption by only 40%.

One of the best times to take part of your supplemental calcium is right before bedtime. This helps keep the body supplied with calcium while you sleep and limits the bone resorption (break down) that normally occurs during the overnight fast.

In a study on the effect of CCM on iron bioavailability, subjects ate a meal containing iron and either took no calcium (the control group) or 500 mg of calcium from either milk, a CCM supplement, or a CCM-fortified beverage.[6] Milk reduced iron absorption by about 60%. The CCM supplement reduced iron absorption by about 25%–30%. *However, iron absorption was normal (not significantly different from the control group) when CCM was given as a fortified beverage.* This fortified beverage contained vitamin C, which helped enhance iron absorption.

Historically, one of the critical studies lacking in this area of calcium-iron interaction was a long-term experiment evaluating the effects of calcium on iron in a population at high risk for iron deficiency. To address this important question, a study was undertaken using CCM as the calcium source and teenage girls as the subject volunteers. Females, during their childbearing years, generally have a greater requirement for iron than males because of blood loss through menstruation. For adolescent girls, the iron is also needed to support growth.

This study was a collaborative effort between Ohio State University and the Procter & Gamble Company.[8] It was funded by the National Institutes of Health, Procter & Gamble, and Ross Products, a division of Abbott Laboratories. For four years, adolescent girls consumed their normal diet and were randomly assigned to either placebo treatment or 1,000 mg of extra calcium per day as a CCM supplement. The average iron intake during the study was 13 mg per day, which corresponds to 87% of the iron RDA. The calcium intakes in the two groups averaged 800 mg for the placebo (calcium from diet only) and 1,600 mg for CCM (diet plus CCM supplement). Following the four years of CCM supplementation, there was no difference between the two groups in blood hemoglobin or hematocrit (clinical measures for iron deficiency anemia). In addition, a special iron-containing protein called ferritin was measured. Ferritin is widely recognized as the single best indicator of long-term total body iron stores. Ferritin acts like a warehouse in your body for storing iron. When people absorb too little iron, their bodies work to maintain hemoglobin and hematocrit levels by pulling iron out from the ferritin warehouse. Thus, when iron is limited, ferritin levels will go down long before any change is seen in hemoglobin and hematocrit levels. *During four years of supplementation with CCM, no changes in ferritin levels were seen. This study clearly established that CCM, even when taken in high amounts, will not interfere with iron.*

Calcium-Magnesium Interaction

It has often been suggested that calcium is capable of blocking magnesium utilization. However, most of this concern is a carry-over from older studies in the nutrition literature. These studies indicated that calcium intakes above 800 mg per day could reduce magnesium balance—that is, more magnesium would be excreted than was being consumed.[5] In essence, this means that calcium could cause a depletion of body magnesium. The more recent studies on calcium-magnesium interaction have produced a mixed bag of results.[4] For example, one study showed that magnesium absorption was reduced by supplementing the diet with 1,700 mg of calcium as calcium gluconate. Another study showed that giving a 1,000-mg dose of calcium as calcium carbonate significantly increased the loss of magnesium in urine. In contrast to these studies, magnesium balance (the net difference between intake and excretion) was unchanged in another study in which calcium intake was increased from 200 mg to 2,000 mg by providing calcium gluconate. Similar results were obtained when 900 mg of calcium was added to the diet either as milk, calcium chloride, or calcium carbonate.

One of the problems in interpreting these studies has been the short duration of the experiments. They have been criticized because increasing calcium intake over a brief time period could produce acute and variable changes in magnesium metabolism. Longer-term studies were needed to allow people to adapt to a high calcium intake before true changes in magnesium absorption could be measured. Thus, we undertook a long-term approach to produce more definitive information about CCM's effect on magnesium utilization.[5] Before any measures of magnesium metabolism were made, subjects received either a placebo or a CCM supplement for 15 weeks. In addition, we stacked the deck in favor of finding a *negative* effect of CCM by increasing calcium intake with CCM by almost 2.5-fold, feeding relatively low amounts of magnesium (only 70% to 75% RDA level), and having rapidly growing adolescent girls serve as subjects.

Following the 15-week adaptation period, the two groups of girls (the placebo group and the CCM-supplemented) came to live at the Ohio State University Clinical Research Facility. Their diets were controlled and supervised for a two-week period, during which magnesium utilization was measured. The two groups consumed the same exact diet, which contained about 700 mg of calcium. This level of calcium was chosen to match the amount the girls had been eating on their own during the 15-week adaptation period. Naturally, the girls who had been taking CCM had a much higher total calcium intake during the prior 15 weeks, about 1,700 mg per day, and this was continued during the magnesium utilization study.

Under these highly monitored conditions, we found absolutely no difference in magnesium utilization between the placebo and CCM groups. Magnesium absorption was the same, magnesium excretion was the same, and magnesium balance was the same.

Calcium-Zinc Interaction

The potentially negative effect of high-calcium diets on zinc utilization is of concern for several reasons. As discussed in Chapter 5, "CCM and Bone Building in Adults," zinc has long been known to participate in normal bone metabolism.[20] Related to this, the combination of zinc, copper, manganese, and CCM is the only multimineral supplement ever shown to completely halt spinal bone loss over a two-year period in postmenopausal women.[21] Normally, the dietary intake of zinc falls well below RDA levels across age groups. In fact, zinc competes strongly with calcium for having the worst intake profile relative to the RDA of any nutrient. Currently, about 73% of all Americans and about 85% of postmenopausal women fall short of the zinc RDA.[17] Zinc deficiency causes loss of appetite, abnormalities in the immune system, and poor growth in children.[22]

Studies dating back almost four decades showed that high calcium diets reduced zinc absorption and brought on signs of zinc deficiency in laboratory animals fed a low zinc-containing diet. Studies in humans have also highlighted the negative impact that high calcium diets can have on zinc. In a study of older men consuming 14 mg of zinc per day (93% RDA), adding calcium gluconate to the diet to raise total calcium intake from about 200 to 900 mg per day cut their zinc absorption in half. Raising the calcium gluconate level to deliver a total of 2,000 mg of calcium essentially brought zinc absorption down to almost zero.[4]

Researchers in the Department of Biochemistry at the University of Sydney, Australia, studied the effects of calcium carbonate and calcium citrate on zinc absorption in young, healthy adult women.[23] The women took a 4.5-mg dose of zinc (38%

RDA) with either no calcium or 600 mg of added calcium as calcium carbonate or calcium citrate. Their increases in blood zinc levels were used to estimate zinc absorption. *Compared to giving zinc alone (with no added calcium), plasma zinc response was reduced by 65% with calcium carbonate and 80% by calcium citrate.*

A study published in 1997 detailed the effects of milk and calcium phosphate on zinc absorption in postmenopausal women.[24] Healthy postmenopausal women, with an average age of 71 years, participated in the study conducted at the USDA Human Nutrition Research Center on Aging at Tufts University. During the study, the women lived in the metabolism research laboratory at the research center and received a controlled diet. The basic diet contained 17.6 mg of zinc (150% RDA) and 900 mg of calcium. Zinc absorption and balance were measured, with or without the addition of an extra 450 mg of calcium supplied as milk or calcium phosphate. *Net zinc absorption was dramatically reduced by both milk and calcium phosphate: It dropped from 13% during the basic diet period (without added calcium) to only 2% when calcium phosphate was added and only 1% when milk was added. The added calcium sources also produced large negative effects on zinc balance.*

A study using similar techniques was conducted on the effects of CCM on zinc absorption and balance in adolescent females.[7] Compared to the study previously mentioned, a greater amount of calcium was given in the form of CCM (1,000 mg of extra calcium per day) and a lower amount of zinc was used in the controlled diet (only 5.5 mg, or 46% of the RDA). These greater calcium and lower zinc levels would presumably magnify any adverse effect of CCM on zinc utilization. *However, no significant negative effect of CCM supplementation on zinc absorption was observed.* The group receiving the basic diet (no CCM added) had a net zinc absorption of 15%, whereas the group taking CCM had a zinc absorption of 21%.

Milk-Alkali Syndrome

Milk-alkali syndrome is a condition historically associated with the consumption of large amounts of calcium in the form of milk combined with "alkali" agents. The alkali agents are antacids such as sodium bicarbonate, and/or calcium, aluminum, or magnesium carbonates or hydroxides. Many years ago physicians commonly tried to manage ulcers by prescribing frequent milk consumption throughout the day, combined with antacids. This practice led to the term *milk-alkali syndrome,* which can have very serious consequences including hypercalcemia (abnormally high blood calcium), lethargy, headache, irritability, memory loss, calcification of soft tissues, kidney damage, and coma.

Milk-alkali syndrome is rarely seen today. However, case study reports occasionally show up in the literature. Drs. Susan Whiting and Richard Wood (University of Saskatchewan and USDA Nutrition Center on Aging) recently reported on 29 cases they found in the literature from 1980 through 1994.[4] Most of the cases (70%) involved a high intake of calcium coupled with some other mitigating circumstance, such as using antacids. However, nine cases were apparently linked to high calcium intake alone. Of these nine cases, the lowest reported calcium intake was 2,000 mg for a five-year period. The calcium intake in the other patients ranged from 3,600–10,800 mg. In the group with mitigating circumstances, the lowest intakes were 2,200–2,500 mg. More typical intakes in these patients were at least 4,000 mg per day and went up as high as 16,500 mg. These case study reports show that in very rare instances, calcium alone, but especially in combination with other risk factors, can be toxic starting at levels as low as 2,000 mg per day. This value is equivalent to drinking slightly less than seven cups of milk or eating about six ounces of hard cheese a day.

Calcium Supplements and Lead

The lead content of calcium supplements is a topic that appears in the popular press from time to time. Usually, the calcium supplements that have been earmarked with a caution about lead are made from bone meal or dolomite. In general, although we all should be cognizant of keeping our lead exposure as low as possible, the highest risk groups for lead toxicity are young children and pregnant women (because of fetal development).

A survey of the lead content of calcium supplement preparations was published in 1993 and, since that time, more attention has been given to the issue.[25] Researchers from Trent University, Ontario, Canada, classified supplements into five types, based on the source of calcium used: bone meal, dolomite, refined calcium carbonate, "fossil shell" calcium carbonate, and calcium chelates. "Fossil shell" calcium carbonate is usually sold as "oyster shell calcium." The calcium chelates would include supplements such as CCM, calcium citrate, calcium lactate, and calcium gluconate. The researchers reported the highest levels of lead in bone meal, fossil shell calcium carbonate, and dolomite supplements. Interestingly, milk was also in the same range, which raises the point that lead intake can also come from our regular food supply. *Calcium chelates and refined calcium carbonate were the lowest in lead.* If you calculate the amount of lead in these products on a mg-for-mg calcium basis, then the sources supplying the most calcium with the least lead are calcium chelates, refined calcium carbonate, and milk. Using the lowest lead-containing sources and sticking with name brand products should increase your margin of safety. However, if you have any doubt, only buy products that list a "1-800" number from the manufacturer somewhere on the package. That way, you can call the company and check whether the products meet federal standards for lead content.

CHAPTER SEVEN

Beyond Healthy Bones— Additional Benefits of Calcium

- Blood Pressure
- Colon Cancer
- Fat and Cholesterol Reduction

In addition to osteoporosis, calcium nutrition has been identified as a possible protective factor in the etiology of high blood pressure and cancer. The link between calcium and these diseases is much less developed than the osteoporosis-calcium connection. As such, the level of consensus surrounding calcium's benefit is weaker and the potential health effects more speculative. Nevertheless, there is at least a hint of calcium's beneficial effect at consumption levels consistent with those needed to ensure optimal bone health. Thus, if you focus on taking calcium for the health of your bones, you may reap additional benefits as well.

Blood Pressure

It has been estimated that as many as 58 million Americans are either taking blood pressure medication and/or have blood pressure high enough to be classified as having Stage 1 hypertension (high blood pressure).[1] The prevalence of hypertension increases with age and is higher in black Americans (38%) than in white Americans (29%).[2] As blood pressure rises out of the normal healthy range, there is an increased risk for heart disease, kidney disease, and stroke. Blood pressure is a function of how vigorously the heart beats, the elasticity of the blood vessels, and the volume and viscosity of blood. The key factor in managing hypertension is early detection. Just as the progression of bone loss and osteoporosis is slow and imperceptible, many people are also unaware that they have elevated blood pressure because there are no overt clinical signs. You should have your blood pressure measured at least every two years, more frequently if you're at increased risk.

Blood pressure readings are normally expressed in units of millimeters of mercury, or mm Hg for short (Hg is the elemental symbol of mercury). Both systolic (the upper number) and diastolic (the lower number) blood pressure can be used to classify blood pressure as normal or high. In the past, more emphasis was given to diastolic blood pressure. It is now clearly recognized that the risk for cardiovascular disease increases with a rise in either systolic or diastolic blood pressure. Thus, the diagnosis of high blood pressure can made based on an above-normal systolic *or* diastolic blood pressure. For adults, "normal" blood pressure is defined as having systolic blood pressure less than 130 mm Hg *and* diastolic blood pressure less than 85 mm Hg. Ideally, these values will be below 120/80 because an increase in risk begins above these levels. So-called "high normal" blood pressure is defined as a systolic value between 130 and 139 and a diastolic value between 85 and 89. Again, although these values fall within the normal range from a definitional point of view, individuals with high normal blood pressure are at increased risk for both fatal and nonfatal cardiovascular events.[1] In addition, once you reach the high normal range, you have a greater chance of developing even higher blood pressure readings.

Stage 1 hypertension is defined by blood pressure readings of 140–159 for systolic and/or 90–99 for diastolic. Stage 2 hypertension values are 160–179/100–109, Stage 3 is 180–209/110–119, and Stage 4 is classified as anything equal to or greater than 210 for systolic and/or equal to or greater than 120 for diastolic. In general, the initial treatment recommended by the National Institutes of Health for Stages 1 or 2 hypertension in otherwise healthy people is modification of lifestyle factors. If the lifestyle changes fail to lower pressure, then the use of antihypertensive medications should be started.[1]

The lifestyle factors that reduce the risk for developing high blood pressure can also lower high blood pressure if you already have it. The factors include body weight reduction, alcohol moderation, regular physical activity, and a reduction in sodium intake. Avoidance of tobacco, although not directly related to blood pressure, is an important adjunct because it reduces the risk for cardiovascular disease, which is strongly linked to high blood pressure. It's interesting to note the substantial overlap in lifestyle factors related to both high blood pressure and osteoporosis. This reinforces the notion that if you maintain a focus on healthy bones, you will reap other health benefits as well.

Body weight above the normal healthy range is closely linked to increases in blood pressure. Conversely, weight reduction alone is highly effective in reducing blood pressure and can increase the effectiveness of anti-hypertensive drugs. In overweight individuals, a loss of as little as 10 pounds can make a difference. Too much alcohol can increase blood pressure and reduce the effectiveness of drug treatments. The upper recommended limit for people with high blood pressure is two drinks per day. Regular physical activity helps reduce high blood pressure and keeps people from developing elevated blood pressure in the first place. Sedentary individuals have a 20% to 50% greater risk of developing high blood pressure.[1] Of course, staying active has other benefits, which include a reduced risk for cardiovascular disease, more effective body weight control, and overall fitness and well-being. Exercise does not need to be particularly vigorous for a blood pressure–lowering benefit. Moderate, but regular, physical activity has been shown to reduce systolic blood pressure by 10 mm Hg.

Dietary sodium intake has been strongly linked to blood pressure. Reducing salt intake to conform to the upper recommended limit (2,300 mg sodium per day) has been shown to produce significant reductions in systolic and diastolic blood pressure. Moreover, a diet that has a healthy amount of sodium (versus a high-sodium diet) may modify other risk factors for hypertension. For example, a study in which sodium was reduced by 2,300 mg per day was shown to curb the typical rise in systolic blood pressure that normally occurs between ages 25 and 55. A reduction in sodium intake by individuals with hypertension reduces blood pressure and can reduce the dosage of medication they need. In some cases, people with Stage 1 hypertension can control blood pressure by doing nothing other than reducing salt intake.[1] In addition to sodium, a number of other dietary elements are linked to blood pressure.

There is evidence that diets high in potassium, and perhaps magnesium, will help keep blood pressure normal. These two elements are found mainly in foods of vegetable origin, whole grains, fruits, vegetables, beans, and so on.

It's interesting to note the substantial overlap in lifestyle factors related to both high blood pressure and osteoporosis. This reinforces the notion that if you maintain a focus on healthy bones, you will reap other health benefits as well.

An interesting dichotomy exists regarding the role of calcium in the control of blood pressure. On one hand, there are data showing an increased risk of developing hypertension when calcium intake is low. On the other hand, increasing blood levels or cellular concentrations of calcium increases blood pressure. In fact, calcium channel–blocker drugs, which block the movement of calcium into cells, are used as antihypertensive agents. These two areas of research, dealing with the benefit of increasing calcium nutrition and the pharmacological benefit of blocking calcium, clearly establish calcium metabolism as a central role player in blood pressure regulation. There is no doubt that calcium metabolism is somehow perturbed during hypertension. However, there is no consensus as to whether this perturbation is the *effect* of high blood pressure or the *cause.* Furthermore, the strength of the data from controlled trials of blood pressure and calcium supplementation varies by the target population studied. Thus, any conclusions regarding the benefit of calcium for maintaining normal blood pressure are tenuous at best. The role of calcium in blood pressure has been investigated in three distinct groups: adults, pregnant women, and children.

Calcium and High Blood Pressure in Adults

The classic study of the relationship between calcium and blood pressure in adults used national survey data to compare dietary calcium intakes to the proportion of individuals with blood pressures falling in the upper 10% of the population. If there is no relationship, then regardless of calcium intake level, 10% of the population at every intake level should be in the upper 10% for blood pressure. The data analysis showed high blood pressure was present in only 4% to 5% of adults with calcium intakes of 1,400 mg per day or more.[3] This percentage was about twice as high for calcium intakes in the 600–800 mg per day range and almost triple at intakes of 200–300 mg. *Several subsequent studies from around the world also found a link between low calcium intake and a risk for high blood pressure.*[3,4] For example, a study from Taiwan showed that consumption of more than 500 mg of calcium per day was significantly more common in men with normal blood pressure than in men with hypertension.[5] A study from Italy showed that consumption of calcium-rich foods was associated with lower blood pressure.[6] From Japan, researchers reported that for each 100-mg increase in calcium consumption, systolic blood pressure was lowered by 0.5 mm Hg.[7]

Additional research indicated that the calcium effect was modified by, or could modify, the impact of other dietary factors. A study known as the Honolulu Heart Study found that men who were moderate to heavy drinkers reaped no blood pressure benefit from diets high in calcium.[8] Another group reported that high sodium and low potassium intakes in the U.S. population were detrimental to blood pressure, but this was only seen in people with a calcium intake below 400 mg per day.[9] These population-based studies of calcium intake and blood pressure were recently reviewed by the Life Sciences Research Office of the Federation of American Societies for Experimental Biology. This group provides scientific assessments of nutrition and medical issues independent of any governmental or nongovernmental groups. They concluded that the population-based studies linking calcium and blood pressure support a possible benefit, especially for groups with low calcium intake.[4]

A better way to isolate the effect of calcium on blood pressure is to conduct controlled studies in which known amounts of extra calcium are given and blood pressure is measured over time. These studies have been done with either calcium supplements or by using diet modification to increase the consumption of calcium-rich foods. One study conducted in the United States tested the effect of 1,000 mg of calcium given as calcium carbonate to men with high normal blood pressure. Following six months of either supplementation or a placebo treatment, no difference in either systolic or diastolic blood pressure was found.[10] A number of other studies have assessed the potential benefit of calcium supplementation and found it to be ineffective. In a study from Italy, researchers reported no difference in blood pressure response to either eight weeks of a placebo or 1,000 mg of calcium in men and women with hypertension.[11] A study from Australia used normal and hypertensive men and women given either a placebo or 400 mg or 800 mg of supplemental calcium in the form of calcium carbonate for two months. No significant difference in blood pressure response was observed in any of the groups.[12] A three-year trial of a placebo versus 1,000 mg of calcium in the form of calcium carbonate plus 1,000 IU of vitamin D in normal men found no effects on blood pressure. Studies in which diet modifications have been made to test blood pressure response to increased calcium intakes have produced mixed results. In one study, factory workers living in New Jersey were asked to increase their calcium intake by 1,150 mg per day by consuming more calcium-rich foods for two months. Compared to the control group, the high-calcium group had a significant decrease of 5 mm Hg in systolic blood pressure.[13] In contrast, a study conducted by researchers at Washington State University showed no difference in blood pressure response when hypertensive male subjects consumed a diet containing 1,500 mg versus 400 mg of calcium per day for four weeks.[14]

The lack of consistency in these studies shows that the effect of increased calcium intake on blood pressure in adults must be very small, if it exists at all. A recent (1997) overall analysis of the calcium and blood pressure scientific literature was conducted by researchers at the National Heart, Lung, and Blood Institute at the National Institutes of Health. After reviewing and analyzing all the studies, the research team concluded that calcium supplementation had no effect on diastolic pressure, caused an average decrease of 0.5 mm Hg in systolic blood pressure in normal people, and led to a 1.7 mm Hg decrease in systolic blood pressure in people with hypertension.[15]

Despite the lack of consistent blood pressure results for increasing calcium intake, per se, there is an indication that low calcium diets may be harmful if the dietary salt intake is high. For example, when people with normal blood pressure were fed a high salt diet with either low (250 mg) or high (2,160) calcium levels, blood pressure went up 9 points in the low calcium group but only 3 points in the high calcium groups.[16] In another study, hypertensive subjects were given a high salt–high calcium diet (1,000 mg of calcium) or a high salt–low calcium diet (400 mg of calcium) for two weeks. Systolic blood pressure went up 14 mm Hg in the low calcium group compared to 7 mm Hg in the high calcium group. Similarly, diastolic blood pressure went up 8 mm Hg in the low calcium group but only 2 mm Hg in the high calcium group.[17] *These studies show that increasing calcium intake can blunt the negative effect of a high salt diet.*

Calcium and High Blood Pressure During Pregnancy

Hypertension during pregnancy is an important public health problem that can be life-threatening to both mother and baby. Hypertension may be present before pregnancy or may develop during pregnancy (pregnancy-induced hypertension). Complications due to hypertension occur in at least 10% of all pregnancies.[2] Pregnancy-induced hypertension is defined as the appearance of blood pressure equal to or greater than 140/90 mm Hg after the 20th week of pregnancy. Several clinical studies have been conducted that demonstrate a benefit of increasing calcium intake on the occurrence of pregnancy-induced hypertension.[4] One of the earlier studies surveyed calcium intake and pregnancy-induced hypertension in women from Canada. The survey showed that the risk of pregnancy-induced hypertension was reduced by 40% in women with the highest (2,300 mg) compared to the lowest (750 mg) calcium intakes.[18] A number of other tests have been conducted to evaluate the effectiveness of calcium supplementation as a way to reduce pregnancy-induced hypertension. In a study conducted in Ecuador, pregnant women at the 24th week of gestation were given either a placebo or 2,000 mg of extra calcium per day in the form of supplemental calcium carbonate. The incidence of pregnancy-induced hypertension was significantly lower in the supplemented versus the placebo group (4% versus 28%).[19] In a similar study from Ecuador, women at high risk for pregnancy-induced hypertension were assigned to either a placebo or 2,000 mg of calcium per day in the form of calcium carbonate. Pregnancy-induced hypertension developed in 71% of the subjects taking the placebo and in only 14% of the women in the calcium supplement group.[20] A study of 1,194 women living in Argentina showed that pregnancy-induced hypertension was reduced by 30% in women receiving 2,000 mg of extra calcium in the form of calcium carbonate beginning at the 20th week of gestation.[21]

These studies show that calcium supplementation can have a positive effect on reducing the risk for pregnancy-induced hypertension, at least in women living in South America. *For women living in the United States the largest (4,600 women) and most recent study (1997) of calcium supplementation (2,000 mg per day) and the risk of pregnancy-induced hypertension revealed no benefit of taking calcium.*[22] Although the prevalence of pregnancy-induced hypertension was 13% greater in the placebo group, this difference was not statistically significant. It is unclear at this time whether ethnic differences and/or differences in the usual dietary calcium intake or other factors account for the lack of consistency in these results from South versus North America.

Calcium and Blood Pressure in Children

Although hypertension can occur during childhood, it is much less common in children than in adults. However, lowering blood pressure within the normal range in children may prevent or postpone the development of hypertension in adulthood. Risk factors for chronic diseases are known to "track" from childhood into adulthood. That is, children who possess the highest values for disease risk factors (such as blood pressure or cholesterol, for example) have the greatest risk of actually developing the disease as adults. This is similar to the theories regarding calcium intake and peak bone mass development in children. Building good peak bone mass during youth will be protective against osteoporotic fractures in later life. With respect to the calcium and hypertension connection, the idea of childhood calcium intake determining risk for the adult onset of hypertension is supported by studies with laboratory animals. A special type of laboratory rat, known as the spontaneously hypertensive rat, or SHR for short, has been used in these experiments. The SHR has normal blood pressure when it's young. However, by five or six weeks of age, it spontaneously develops elevated blood pressure. A number of studies have shown that high dietary calcium will reduce the rise in blood pressure in the SHR. Conversely, calcium restriction in the SHR causes the blood pressure to rise even higher than it normally would.[4]

To address the potential for this to occur in humans, a study was conducted on the effects of CCM supplementation on blood pressure in children.[23] This was a collaborative effort between Boston University and the Procter & Gamble Company, with most of the funding for the study coming from the National Institutes of Health. One hundred and one, male and female, fifth-grade students (average age 11 years) attending a public elementary school in Boston agreed to participate. The majority of the participants were black Americans. There is a special interest in calcium's potential to control the blood pressure of black Americans. Compared to white Americans, they typically have lower calcium intakes and higher rates of hypertension.[2]

The children were randomly assigned to receive a CCM-fortified beverage or an identical-looking and -tasting beverage without CCM for a 12-week period. Throughout the study, the children, their teachers and parents, and the study investigators were denied knowledge of the identity of the beverages. Each day the students drank two 8-ounce beverage servings supplying either zero calcium (the placebo) or 600 mg of calcium (CCM). On school days, the beverages were consumed while at school. On the weekends, the students took the beverages home to drink. No other changes to the children's diets were made. A detailed analysis of their usual diets showed no differences in sodium (3,200 mg per day) or calcium intakes (860 mg per day).

Blood pressure was measured at the beginning, midpoint, and end of the 12-week period. In addition, blood pressure was measured six weeks after CCM supplementation was stopped. Blood pressure was monitored very carefully during the study by taking four separate readings at each setting with an automated measuring device. The effect of CCM supplementation on blood pressure was significant and depended on the amount of calcium the children usually consumed. CCM reduced systolic blood pressure by 3.5 mm Hg in children with the lowest quartile (lowest one-fourth) of calcium intake (565 mg per day). The second quartile of calcium intake (755 mg) had a blood pressure–lowering effect from CCM of 2.8 mm Hg. The third quartile (915 mg) reduced blood pressure by 1.3 mm Hg, and the fourth quartile (1,190 mg) showed no effect. The differences in blood pressure between the CCM and placebo groups disappeared six weeks after CCM supplementation was stopped. *This study shows that blood pressure can be lowered in children by increasing their calcium intake.* The greatest effect is seen in children with the lowest calcium intakes, and if supplementation is stopped, the blood pressure benefit is not maintained.

Colon Cancer

According to the American Cancer Society, colon cancer is the second leading cause of death from cancer after lung cancer. About equal numbers of men and women die each year from colon cancer in the United States. A number of dietary factors are postulated to be related to colon cancer risk, including the excessive intake of fat, and the lack of fiber, fruits and vegetables, and vitamin D in the American diet. The role of calcium in the etiology of colon cancer has been investigated, using a number of experimental models. *In vitro (test tube) experiments, controlled studies of laboratory animals and humans, and population-based studies have all demonstrated a positive effect of increased calcium intake on decreasing the risk of colon cancer.*[24–28]

One of the important markers for cancer risk that has been used in animal and human studies is the hyperproliferation (rapid growth of new cells) of precancerous cells lining the intestinal tract.[28] Increased proliferation of the cells in the intestinal tract is one of the earliest changes seen during the eventual development of cancer. Although hyper-proliferation occurs all the time, the more it occurs and the more it is allowed to proceed unchecked, the greater the risk of it progressing to a cancerous stage. A number of studies with laboratory rodents have shown that high dietary calcium intake will decrease hyper-proliferation and, in some cases, tumor occurrence, in animals given cancer-inducing agents.[28]

Colon cancer risk was reduced by 60% in men consuming 1,400 mg of calcium or more. For women, the risk of colon cancer was 50% lower in those consuming 600 mg of calcium or more.

Related studies in humans have shown the same type of calcium effect. For example, a study reported in the *New England Journal of Medicine* found that supplementation with 1,250 mg of calcium to individuals with a family history of colon cancer significantly reduced hyper-proliferation.[29] Another human study involved individuals who had previously undergone the removal of colonic adenomas. Adenomas are benign tumors that are believed to represent an intermediate stage between normal intestinal cells and cancer. Subjects who received 1,500 mg of supplemental calcium for 90 days showed a 23% reduction in the proliferative activity of cells taken from a rectal biopsy.[30] In a similar study, subjects given 2,000 mg of supplemental calcium for 30 days showed a 31% reduction in proliferative activity.[30] In a third study, the same type of subjects received either a placebo or 2,000 mg of supplemental calcium for four weeks, then switched treatments for an additional four weeks. Proliferative activity was significantly reduced only during the supplementation phase.[30]

A number of population-based studies also support the notion that greater intakes of calcium will reduce the risk for colon cancer. For example, researchers from the University of California, San Diego, reported on the incidence of colon cancer in 1,954 men over a 19-year period. The highest incidence of colon cancer occurred in men with the lowest calcium intake, 300–750 mg per day. Colon cancer risk was reduced by 40% in men consuming between 750 and 1,200 mg of calcium, and by 70% in those consuming greater than 1,200 mg of calcium.[27] They also found a significant effect of vitamin D intake on risk. Men with intakes of 230 IU of vitamin D or greater had a 50% reduction in colon cancer risk compared to men consuming less. Researchers from the University of Utah Medical School conducted a study of both men and women ages 40 to 79, in which the dietary calcium intakes of colon cancer patients and control subjects were documented over a three-year period. The results were similar to those found in the previous study: An inverse relationship was observed between colon cancer risk and calcium intake. Men consuming between 975 and 1,400 mg of calcium were 20% less likely to develop colon cancer than those consuming less. Colon cancer risk was reduced by 60% in men consuming 1,400 mg of calcium or more. For women, the risk of colon cancer was 50% lower in those consuming 600 mg of calcium or more.[26]

Although long-term supplementation trials of calcium, either alone or in combination with vitamin D, and its effect on colon cancer have not been performed, the data from animal studies, short-term studies of hyperproliferation in high-risk patients, and the positive findings from population-based studies show a promising calcium-based approach for controlling colon cancer. Moreover, the levels of calcium intake at which benefits start to be seen (1,000–1,500 mg) are consistent with those needed to ensure optimal bone health.

Fat and Cholesterol Reduction

Coronary heart disease is the leading cause of death in the United States, accounting for at least 1.25 million heart attacks and about 500,000 deaths each year.[2] Although there are many related causes for coronary heart disease, three major risk factors—high blood pressure, cigarette smoking, and high blood cholesterol levels—can be modified through lifestyle choices. Diet can play a major role in regulating both blood pressure and blood cholesterol levels. A widespread body of evidence shows that the risk for coronary heart disease increases as blood cholesterol levels increase. Similar to the association between blood pressure and heart attacks, even blood cholesterol levels in the "normal" range are linked to increased risk for developing coronary heart disease. Average cholesterol levels in adults are generally in the range of 210 to 215 mg per deciliter (mg/dl) of blood. A desirable level is considered less than 200 mg/dl, although risk for coronary heart disease may increase when values begin to rise above 180 mg/dl.[2] Cholesterol values between 200 and 239 mg/dl are considered borderline high, and individuals with levels at or above 240 mg/dl are considered to have high blood cholesterol (hypercholesterolemia). In particular, increased levels of LDL cholesterol, the so-called "bad cholesterol," accounts for most of the increased risk for coronary heart disease when total cholesterol levels are high.

The most potent cause of blood cholesterol level is saturated fat.[31] Although dietary cholesterol can also raise blood cholesterol levels, its impact is much weaker than that of saturated fat. Given the strong relationship among saturated fat, blood cholesterol levels, and increased risk for developing coronary heart disease, a number of public health agencies have recommended the reduction of fat intake in the diet, particularly saturated fat. Typical recommendations call for no more than 30% of your total calories from fat, with no more than 10% coming from saturated fat.[31]

Another approach to reducing the effect of saturated fat in the diet on blood cholesterol levels would be to reduce its absorption. Normally, humans are very efficient at absorbing fat, averaging about 95% to 99% absorption.[31] The fat in the diet usually comes in as a triglyceride, which is composed of three fatty acid molecules chemically bound to one molecule of glycerol. Before the fatty acids can be absorbed, they are cleaved from the glycerol molecule. These "free fatty acids" are vulnerable to complexing with other materials in the intestine that can reduce their absorption. One of the materials that has this effect is calcium. The calcium–fatty acid complex is very insoluble and thus precipitates in the intestine and cannot be absorbed.

To test the potential of CCM supplementation to reduce saturated fat absorption and blood cholesterol levels, a study was undertaken with a group of men who had borderline hypercholesterolemia (high blood cholesterol levels).[32] The men were between the ages of 38 and 49 and in good general health (except for their cholesterol levels). In random order, they were fed two different test diets. Both diets mimicked a typical American diet, with 34% of the total calories coming from total fat and 13% from saturated fat. The cholesterol content of the diets was the same, 240 mg per day. The only difference between the diets was the addition of CCM. The control diet (without CCM) contained 400 mg of calcium. The high-calcium diet contained an extra 1,800 mg of calcium supplied as CCM, to bring the total calcium content up to 2,200 mg per day. The CCM was provided as a combination of supplement tablets, a beverage, and CCM-fortified muffins. All of the subjects consumed both diets during two separate 10-day periods.

Thus, the use of calcium supplementation and calcium-fortified foods can be an effective approach for augmenting efforts to lower blood cholesterol levels and decrease saturated fat absorption.

Compared to the control diet, *the CCM-fortified diet resulted in a twofold increase in saturated fat excretion. In addition, total blood cholesterol was reduced with CCM by 6% and LDL cholesterol was reduced by 11%*. This magnitude of cholesterol lowering is similar to what has been found using soluble fibers. For example, in a recent study (1998) of the effects of psyllium husk, the addition of three servings of psyllium-containing foods (cereals, bread, pasta, or snack bars) reduced LDL cholesterol by 5%.[33] This amount of psyllium is about equal to three doses of a psyllium-based bulk fiber laxative. Other studies have shown that the addition of three servings of oatmeal per day to the diet will reduce LDL cholesterol by 10%.[34] Thus, the use of calcium supplementation and calcium-fortified foods can be an effective approach for augmenting efforts to lower blood cholesterol levels and decrease saturated fat absorption.

CHAPTER EIGHT

The Best Sources of Dietary Calcium

- **Calcium Content**
- **Frequency of Consumption**
- **Calcium Absorption**
- **Cost**
- **Putting It All Together**
- **How Can I Tell If I'm Getting Enough Calcium?**

There are four main factors determining the potential usefulness of a food (or beverage) as a source of dietary calcium:

1. Calcium content
2. Calcium bioavailability (absorption)
3. Expected frequency of consumption
4. Cost

The cost factor is generally a minor concern because you need to eat anyway and there really aren't any exotic/expensive foods that offer advantages for supplying calcium. Furthermore, the foods with the highest calcium content tend to supply the most calcium at the lowest cost on a mg-calcium-per-dollar basis. However, another way to look at the cost of calcium is the number of calories a food contains relative to its calcium content, the "caloric cost" of calcium. You only have so many calories to spend each day, so you need to spend them wisely.

The triad of other factors, calcium content, bioavailability, and frequency of consumption, are the foundation principles for designing a diet that meets optimal intake recommendations. If any one of these factors is weak, you won't be able to achieve the desired result. Consuming a diet that supplies the optimal amount of calcium exclusively from foods naturally rich in calcium is certainly achievable. However, it isn't very probable. Current intakes of calcium fall so far short of optimal that major changes in dietary behaviors and food patterns are required. The use of fortified foods and supplements provide the added flexibility that most people need to achieve the optimal intake levels. The use of fortified foods and supplements has not been overtly recommended by public health agencies. However, they have recognized their potential usefulness and have, in effect, given people permission to incorporate them into an overall healthy diet.

In this chapter, I'll put the four factors determining the usefulness of dietary calcium sources into perspective for you. Then we'll put it all together to come up with your best approach for meeting optimal calcium intake recommendations.

Calcium Content

The calcium content of foods varies widely, covering a range that spans zero mg of calcium, all the way up to several hundred mg per serving. The easiest way to look at the calcium content of foods in relationship to an overall healthy diet is to examine foods comprising the USDA's Food Guide Pyramid to see how each of the six food groups stacks up. Although there is some variability in the calcium content of different foods within each group, I've selected representative and common food items to make it easy to see relative differences among the groups.

The foundation group of the Food Guide Pyramid (i.e., the group you should eat the most servings from) is breads, cereals, rice, grains, and pasta. The USDA recommends we consume 6 to 11 servings per day from this group, depending on our caloric need. In general, these foods are low in fat, low in calories, and low in calcium. Although breakfast cereals are commonly fortified with several vitamins and minerals, calcium is usually not one of them. For example, the average calcium content of a one-ounce serving of Corn Flakes, Grapes Nuts, Raisin Bran, Puffed Rice, and Shredded Wheat is 7 mg. In addition, since grains have so little calcium, it doesn't matter much if you use whole grains or their more highly processed counterparts. For example one-half cup of white rice has 2 mg of calcium and brown rice has 10 mg. A one-ounce serving (one slice) of whole wheat bread has 24 mg of calcium; white bread also has 24 mg. Taking into account a wide range of cereal and grain products, including breads, hot cereals, cold cereals, crackers, pastas, and different grains, the average calcium content of a serving from this food group supplies 10 mg of calcium.[1] Thus, your 6–11 recommended servings per day equates to about 60–110 mg of calcium.

The next two groups in the Food Guide Pyramid are the vegetable group and fruit group. The recommended number of servings per day from these groups are three to five vegetables and two to four fruits. Whole fruits and vegetables form an important part of any overall healthy diet. A great many population-based studies have shown that people who eat lots of fruits and vegetables have significantly lower risks for a number of chronic diseases. According to the National Cancer Institute, a balanced diet that is high in fruits and vegetables and low in fat will lower your risk for several types of cancer. They recommend that you eat at least five total servings per day (fruits and vegetables combined).

Fruits and vegetables are generally low in fat, low in calories, and low in calcium. To calculate an average value for the calcium content of vegetables, I used the following: asparagus, broccoli, carrots, celery, corn, green beans, peas, mushrooms, onions, green peppers, potatoes, tomatoes, and zucchini. The average calcium content for a one-half cup serving is 12 mg.[1] Some vegetables have a higher calcium content; broccoli contains 21 mg of calcium per one-half cup. But most people don't exclusively eat broccoli as their only vegetable source. In fact, potatoes (mainly French fried) are the most popular vegetable in United States and contain only 3 mg of calcium per one-half cup. On average, if you consume the recommended three to five servings of vegetables per day, your calcium intake from this food group will be 36–60 mg.

I used the following items to calculate an average calcium value for the fruit group: apples, oranges, bananas, pears, peaches, grapes, strawberries, pineapple, cantaloupe, and watermelon. A serving size in this case was one piece of fruit (except for pineapple, watermelon, and cantaloupe for which I used one cup), or one cup of grapes or strawberries. The average calcium value of these fruits is 17 mg, according to values published in the USDA's handbook on the composition of foods.[1] Thus, the two to four recommended servings of fruit from the Food Guide Pyramid will supply an average of about 34–68 mg. Combine this with the contribution of the vegetable group and you get a range of 70–128 mg of calcium, going from the lowest to the highest recommended number of servings.

The meat group in the Food Guide Pyramid is actually composed of meat, poultry, fish, eggs, beans, and nuts, all potential sources of protein in the diet. The fat and calorie content of these foods varies dramatically, but their calcium contents are all low. For example, a one-half cup serving of lima beans (3 ounces) has 27 mg of calcium and 0 grams of fat. Compare that to a 3-ounce serving of broiled lean ground beef, which has 9 mg of calcium and 16 grams of fat. Chicken, pork, and fish also have very low levels of calcium, less than 20–25 mg per 3-ounce portion. An egg contains 25 mg of calcium. Nuts average about 30 mg per 1-ounce serving. One exception to the low calcium content of the "protein food group" is canned fish. The trick here is that you need to eat the bones found in canned salmon and sardines (tuna doesn't have them). Three ounces of sardines has 372 mg of calcium and salmon contains 167 mg (per 3 ounces). The overall average calcium content for this food group (excluding canned fish with bones) is about 25 mg, with beans, nuts, and eggs being the highest sources. If you consume the recommended two to three servings per day, you should obtain 50–75 mg of calcium.

As a group, foods that the USDA recommends we should eat sparingly (fats, oils, and sweets) contain very little, if any, calcium. That's because sugar and fat don't have calcium. These foods include table sugar, honey, cooking oil, butter, shortening, candy, or foods containing large amounts of sugar and/or fat.

Before we move on to dairy products and calcium-fortified foods, let's total up the calcium supplied from all the other food groups. Remember, there is range of servings per day recommended for each group, which depends on caloric need. The greater number of serving sizes are obviously for larger individuals or, more appropriately, for those who burn more calories through physical activity at their jobs or by exercising. The range of calcium intake supplied by all the food groups combined is between 180 and 313 mg per day. Thus, assuming you don't eat many fatty or highly sugared products but rather, consume the recommend amounts of the healthy foods contained in Food Guide Pyramid, you can expect a diet completely devoid of dairy, fortified foods, or supplements to supply about 200–300 mg of calcium per day.

Given the previous contribution of calcium from the other food groups, it's easy to see why so many women fall far short of the recommended calcium intakes of 1,000–1,500 mg per day. Without the use of dairy products, calcium-fortified foods, and/or supplements, you have no chance of coming anywhere near this optimal range. Within the dairy group, your basic choices are milk, cheese, and yogurt. The calcium content of milk is fairly consistent, regardless of fat content, and a good working average is 300 mg per 8 ounces. Yogurt varies quite a bit in calcium, depending on the type and serving size. Most people like yogurt with fruit added, which lowers the calcium content by diluting the yogurt. Moreover, the container size for single serving yogurts can vary anywhere from 4 to 8 ounces. The overall average calcium content for low-fat, fruited varieties of yogurt is about 300 mg per 8 ounces. The calcium content of cheeses varies all over the map. Soft cheeses such as cream cheese and cottage cheese are very low in calcium, only 20–25 mg per ounce. The calcium contents of 1 ounce of some of the most popular cheeses are: Swiss—272 mg, Cheddar—204 mg, American—174 mg, and mozzarella (frequently used on pizza)—147 mg. A good working average for these common cheeses is about 200 mg per ounce.

The Food Guide Pyramid recommends two to three serving of dairy products per day, which would supply between 600–900 mg of calcium (a serving equals one cup of milk or yogurt, or 1.5 ounces of cheese). Combine this with the calcium contribution from the other food groups (200–300 mg) and you have a range of calcium intakes, depending on the number of servings, that goes from 800–1,200 mg per day. Thus, if you consume the maximum number of servings per day from the Food Guide Pyramid (roughly equivalent to a 2,800-calorie diet), and choose the richest sources of dairy calcium, then it is possible to approach the optimal level for calcium intake. Needless to say, this type of diet represents a very uncommon occurrence in America, let alone in most other parts of the world, where dairy product consumption is not practiced. Thus, it's not surprising that nearly *100%* of all women ages 51 or older fail to consume the recommended amount of calcium. Men in this age group don't do much better, with approximately 90%–95% falling short.[2]

The landscape for calcium-fortified foods is difficult to dimension because it's in an early stage of evolution with new product introductions very likely to occur. Products with the longest history in the marketplace are fortified beverages such as orange juice and Sunny Delight with Calcium. These beverages contain 300–350 mg of calcium per 8-ounce serving, equivalent to the calcium content of milk. In addition, a number of dairy products with added calcium have been recently introduced, including calcium-fortified milk, yogurt, cottage cheese, and frozen yogurt. These products generally contain 33%–100% more calcium than their unfortified counterparts. Although these products contain more calcium per serving, they are unlikely to increase the number of servings of dairy products consumed. For example, the calcium content of fortified milk has been enhanced from 300 to 500 mg per 8-ounce serving. However, the average total milk consumption by adult women is only 4.5 ounces per day.[3] Thus, switching from regular to calcium-fortified milk will boost the total calcium intake derived from milk from 170 to 280 mg per day. Although this is a helpful increase, it hardly closes the gap between our current low calcium intake and the optimal amount. Calcium-fortified cottage cheese has twice the amount of the unfortified version. However, it is relatively low in calcium to begin with (20 mg versus 40 mg per ounce in the fortified brands) and very few people eat it on a regular basis. These examples bring us to the second factor that determines the usefulness of a dietary calcium source, frequency of consumption.

Frequency of Consumption

To be of value as a calcium source, a food must be both high in calcium and consumed on a frequent basis. A good example of this is the relative contribution of grain products (bread, rolls, crackers, pasta, and cereals) to the total supply of calcium in our diets. Most Americans consume some type of grain product (usually several servings) every day. In fact, the average number of servings is about 6.5 per day. However, because of their very low calcium content, grains typically account for only 5% of the total calcium consumed in the American diet. In contrast, dairy products, which have a much lower frequency of consumption but a higher calcium content, contribute about 75% of the total calcium consumed. On an individual basis, you need to find a food (or foods) rich in calcium that you like well enough to consume every day in quantities sufficient to supply 900–1,200 mg per day. This intake, when combined with the calcium that comes from the rest of your diet, should put you in the optimal calcium intake range. It is unlikely that any fruit, vegetable, meat, or grain product will meet this requirement. I don't care how many times broccoli gets recommended as a "good" source of calcium, no one is going to eat 21 cups of broccoli per day (this would supply 900 mg of calcium). Even if you did like broccoli well enough to eat this huge amount, it obviously would leave little room for other foods and certainly does not represent a well-balanced, varied diet. Thus, the frequent consumption of dairy foods, calcium-fortified foods, and/or the use of calcium supplements is the only practical approach for most people to successfully consume calcium within the optimal intake range.

Calcium Absorption

To help keep your skeleton strong, the calcium you eat must be absorbed. Calcium absorption varies widely (about tenfold) from different sources, especially among foods. This topic is covered in detail in Chapter 2. But let's run through some of the basics of absorption as it relates to the food groups in the Food Guide Pyramid, calcium-fortified foods, and supplements.

Studies with whole wheat bread have shown calcium absorption to be about equivalent to the calcium from milk.[4]

Little research has been conducted on the calcium absorption from other grain products. Even less work has been done regarding the calcium in fruits. However, since they generally lack any constituent known to block calcium absorption, there is no reason to suspect that calcium from fruits will be less well-absorbed than calcium in milk. Flesh foods (meat, poultry, fish) contribute so little calcium to our diet that absorption is practically a moot point. The exception to this is canned fish with bones. Although the calcium absorption from fish bones has not been measured, calcium absorption tests have been done on ground-up cow bones and calcium phosphate (which resembles bones in composition). These studies show calcium absorption that is about 30% less than milk.[5] Similarly, the calcium in nuts and beans has been found to be 35%–50% less well-absorbed than the calcium in milk.[6]

The calcium absorption from many vegetables is generally as good as, if not better, than milk. One exception to this is spinach, which has a calcium absorption approximately 80%–90% lower than milk.[7,8] On the other end of the spectrum, cruciferous vegetables tend to be some of the most concentrated sources of vegetable calcium and have calcium absorption that exceeds that of milk. The average calcium absorption from a serving of broccoli, brussels sprouts, cauliflower, or kale is about 90% greater than the calcium from milk.[6] Unfortunately, although these foods are high in calcium as far as vegetables are concerned, they have very little calcium compared to milk or CCM-fortified beverages. On a serving-for-serving basis, they only contain about 10% of the calcium in milk or CCM beverages. Therefore, even with their high absorption figured into the equation, you would need to eat about six servings of cruciferous vegetables to get the same amount of absorbable calcium that is in one glass of milk and about nine servings to equal one glass of a CCM-fortified beverage.

On an individual basis, you need to find a food (or foods) rich in calcium that you like well enough to consume every day in quantities sufficient to supply 900–1,200 mg per day. This intake, when combined with the calcium that comes from the rest of your diet, should put you in the optimal calcium intake range.

With the exception of CCM-fortified beverages, the absorption of calcium from calcium-fortified foods has not been well documented. However, these products are fortified with the same calcium sources used in calcium supplements (usually calcium phosphate, calcium carbonate, or calcium lactate). Thus, the absorption from the fortified fraction of these foods is presumably equivalent to their absorption in supplemental (tablet) form. One food (other than CCM products) that has been assessed and found to be equivalent to milk is calcium-set tofu (contains calcium sulfate).[6]

The calcium absorption from milk, yogurt, and cheese is known to be equivalent.[9] In addition, several studies have shown that milk and calcium carbonate supplements yield the same percentage of calcium absorption.[9–11] Furthermore, a study published in the *New England Journal of Medicine* shows that calcium absorption is the same from milk, calcium carbonate, calcium citrate, calcium lactate, and calcium gluconate.[11] In contrast to these findings, the absorption of calcium from CCM supplements and CCM-fortified beverages has been repeatedly documented to exceed the absorption of calcium from milk and calcium carbonate by at least 30% and up to 50%.[6,10,12–14] This high absorption of calcium from CCM has been shown in children, young adults, and postmenopausal women. In addition, on an ounce-for-ounce basis, CCM-fortified beverages contain as much calcium as milk. Thus, they provide a greater amount of absorbable calcium per serving than milk.

Cost

Cost, per se, should not be a significant consideration in determining the usefulness of a calcium source. Irrespective of your calcium intake, you need to purchase food, and none of the significantly rich sources of calcium are cost-prohibitive. However, it is interesting to compare the dollar cost of obtaining calcium from different foods to emphasize the point that dairy products and calcium-fortified foods are the most valuable choices, both in terms of calcium content and economy. For comparison, I've selected products that represent the richest calcium sources in their respective food groups. The cost numbers I used simply reflect prices found on a given day in my local grocery store (in Cincinnati, Ohio). Thus, they don't necessarily represent national averages. However, the cost differences between products should generally reflect relative differences you will find in your own hometown or city. Because many people are interested in reducing the fat content in their diet, I've also included the amount of fat that comes from these products. See Table 8-1 for the cost and fat content of foods that supply 300 mg of calcium. Although they are not included in the table, calcium supplements supply calcium at a lower cost than any food and obviously contain no fat.

On an ounce-for-ounce basis, CCM-fortified beverages contain as much calcium as milk. Thus, they provide a greater amount of absorbable calcium per serving than milk.

Putting It All Together

Using the Food Guide Pyramid is a good yardstick to measure the overall healthfulness of your diet. It parallels the recommendations of several public health organizations for a diet

Table 8-1 Cost and Fat Content of Foods That Supply 300 mg of Calcium

Food Item	Amount	Cost ($)	Fat (grams)
Milk—2%	8 ounces	$0.15	4.7
Sunny Delight with Calcium (CCM)	8 ounces	$0.20	0.0
Tropicana Pure Premium with Calcium (CCM)	7 ounces	$0.32	0.0
Cheddar Cheese	1.5 ounces	$0.45	14.0
Yogurt—low fat, fruited	1 cup	$0.79	3.0
Pinto Beans—canned, no fat	3.5 cups	$0.86	0.0
Whole Wheat Bread	13 slices	$1.12	12.5
Cottage Cheese—2%	2 cups	$1.28	8.7
Almonds—dry roasted	3.75 ounces	$1.87	56.0
Broccoli	7 cups	$2.09	0.0
Sardines—water packed	2.5 ounces	$2.09	18.0
Grape Nuts Cereal	7 cups	$4.62	15.0
Strawberries	15 cups	$8.25	0.0

that promotes good health and reduces risk of disease. The Food Guide Pyramid emphasizes the consumption of complex carbohydrates from grain products (especially whole grains), lots of fruits and vegetables, low-fat dairy products, legumes, lean cuts of meat, and limited intakes of fat, oil, and sweets.

Although very sound in its overall approach for achieving a healthy, well-balanced diet, the problem with the Food Guide

Pyramid when it comes to calcium is that you need to consume the maximum number of serving amounts to have any hope of coming close to optimal intake recommendations. Furthermore, when you look at the caloric content of sample diets constructed from the Food Guide Pyramid, the higher number of servings from the various food groups correspond with a diet containing about 2,800 calories.[15] In general, this caloric intake would only be appropriate for teenage boys, physically active men, and very physically active women. The lower-to-middle range of the serving amounts, from which it is essentially impossible to achieve the optimal calcium intake, corresponds to a caloric intake (1,600–2,200 calories) appropriate for older men and women, all sedentary or moderately active younger women, most children, teenage girls, and sedentary men.[15] A further challenge is that many people are consuming a diet that more closely resembles an "inverted pyramid"—that is, foods at the narrow top of the pyramid, which should be consumed in limited quantities (fats, oils, sweets), comprise a large proportion of our total caloric intake. The combination of added sugars and "discretionary fat" intake comprise about 40% of the total calories in the typical American diet.[15] Discretionary fats are those you either add to food or eat by virtue of selecting a high-fat version of foods when lower-fat versions are available. Examples of this include spreading cream cheese on a bagel or eating French fries instead of a baked potato or rice.

To address the calcium issue in the context of an overall healthy diet, you need to do one of three things (or use a combination approach). First, you need to become more physically active so you can eat more. Second, each day you need to incorporate three to four servings of low-fat dairy products and/or calcium-fortified foods or beverages into your diet. For most of you, this will mean the addition of two to three servings on top of what you already eat. Third, if you can't find calcium-rich foods (dairy or fortified) that fit into your daily diet, then start using a calcium supplement.

How Can I Tell If I'm Getting Enough Calcium?

There isn't any blood test you can take to tell if your calcium is adequate or deficient. That's because calcium concentrations in the blood are very tightly controlled regardless of your calcium intake. In fact, the high degree of blood calcium regulation is one of the main reasons bones become weaker when calcium intake is inadequate. Calcium is essential to the normal functioning of virtually every cell in the body, not just bones. It is intimately involved with processes of muscle contraction, nerve transmission, blood vessel constriction or dilation, secretions from glands, blood clotting, communication within cells in response to hormones, and so on. Calcium's pivotal role in metabolism causes our bodies to precisely control blood calcium levels within a narrow range. The control of blood calcium concentration is so important that our bodies readily take calcium out of the skeleton to maintain blood levels when our calcium intake is too low.

Bone density measurements are extremely useful for assessing the health of the skeleton, and I urge you to have your bone density measured. Bone density is strongly related to bone strength and is predictive of fracture risk. However, bone density, per se, is not an indication of the adequacy of calcium intake. Genetics and a number of environmental factors other than calcium affect bone density. Thus, it can't be used as a reliable guide for assessing calcium intake. Besides, even if your bone density is high for your age, you want to keep it that way, which means optimizing calcium intake and other lifestyle factors related to bone health. Similar to bone density, urine calcium levels are affected by a host of other factors other than calcium intake and are an unreliable indicator of dietary intake.

Since there is no biochemical test or physical measurement that reflects the adequacy of calcium intake, the only way to ensure you're getting enough is to become familiar with the calcium content of foods/beverages and supplements and be sure to consume the recommended amounts.

Since there is no biochemical test or physical measurement that reflects the adequacy of calcium intake, the only way to ensure you're getting enough is to become familiar with the calcium content of foods/beverages and supplements and be sure to consume the recommended amounts. To reiterate, these are 800–1,200 mg for children, 1,200–1,500 mg for adolescents and young adults, 1,000 mg for adults, and 1,200–1,500 mg for anyone over 50 years of age. It's possible that your own individual optimal calcium intake (the amount at which you maximize the calcium benefit) is below these recommended levels. However, there is no test you can take to be sure. Thus, if you want to ensure the maximum benefit, you need to consume 100% of the optimal amount of calcium. In addition, the intelligent selection of calcium sources such as CCM, which have high bioavailability and proven effectiveness for bone, will further serve to guarantee your own personal optimal bone health.

Notes

Chapter One

1. Food and Nutrition Board, Institute of Medicine. "Dietary Reference Intakes: Calcium, Phosphorus, Magnesium, Vitamin D, and Fluoride." (Washington, DC: National Academy Press, 1997).
2. Ray NF, Chan JK, Thamer M, Melton LJ. "Medical Expenditures for the Treatment of Osteoporotic Fractures in the United States in 1995: Report from the National Osteoporosis Foundation." *J Bone Miner Res* (1997); 12: 24–35.
3. Johnston CC Jr, Melton LJ, Lindsay R, Eddy DM. "Clinical Indications for Bone Mass Measurements: A Report from the Scientific Advisory Board of the National Osteoporosis Foundation." *J Bone Miner Res* (1989); 4 (suppl. 2): 1–27.
4. Wilson JW, Wilkinson-Enns C, Goldman JD, Tippett KS, Mickle SJ, Cleveland LE, Chahil PS. "Combined Results from USDA's 1994 and 1995 Continuing Survey of Food Intakes by Individuals and 1994 and 1995 Diet and Health Knowledge Survey." Department of Agriculture, Agricultural Research Service, Beltsville Human Nutrition Research Center, Food Surveys' Research Group (Riverdale, MD: 1997).

5. NIH Consensus Development Panel on Optimal Calcium Intake. "NIH Consensus Conference: Optimal Calcium Intake." *JAMA* (1994); 272: 1942–48.
6. Robertson WG. "Chemistry and Biochemistry of Calcium." In *Calcium in Human Biology*, ed. BEC Nordin (University Printing House Oxford: Springer-Verlag, 1988), 1–26.
7. Eaton SB, Neson DA. "Calcium in Evolutionary Perspective." *Am J Clin Nutr* (1991); 54: 281S–87S.
8. Houts SS. "Lactose Intolerance." *Food Technology 1988;* (March issue): 110–13.
9. Coelho AM, Bramblett CA, Quick LB, Branblett SS. "Resource Availability and Population Density in Primates: A Socio-Bioenergetic Analysis of Energy Budgets of Guatemalan Howler and Spider Monkeys." *Primates* (1976); 17: 63–80.
10. Eaton SB, Konner M. "Paleolithic Nutrition: A Consideration of Its Nature and Current Implications." *N Engl J Med* (1985); 312: 283–89.
11. Department of Health, Education, and Welfare. *Dietary Intake Source Data United States, 1971–74* (National Center for Health Statistics, 1979) [DHEW publication (PHS) No. 79–1221].
12. Schneider EL, Guralnik JM. "The Aging of America: Impact on Health Care Costs." *JAMA* (1990); 263: 2335–40.
13. United States Department of Agriculture, Human Nutrition Information Service. "Composition of Foods." *Agricultural Handbooks No. 8–1 through 8–20* (Washington, DC: U.S. Government Printing Office, 1976–1989).
14. Heaney RP, Weaver CM, Recker RR. "Calcium Absorption from Spinach." *Am J Clin Nutr* (1988); 47: 707–09.
15. Weaver CM, Plawecki KL. "Dietary Calcium: Adequacy of a Vegetarian Diet." *Am J Clin Nutr* (1994); 59 (suppl.): 1238S–41S.
16. Andon MB, Peacock M, Kanerva RL, De Castro JAS. "Calcium Absorption from Apple and Orange Juice Fortified with Calcium Citrate Malate (CCM)." *J Am Coll Nutr* (1996); 15: 313–16.

17. Andon M, Kanerva R, Cummins S, Luhrsen K, Chatzidakis C, Smith K. "Calcium Bioavailability from Calcium Salts, Milk, and Juice Drinks Fortified with Calcium Citrate Malate." *FASEB J* (1993); 7: A308.
18. Smith KT, Heaney RP, Flora L, Hinders SM. "Calcium Absorption from a New Calcium Delivery System (CCM)." *Calcif Tissue Int* (1987); 41: 351–52.
19. Miller JZ, Smith DL, Flora L, Slemenda C, Jiang X, Johnston CC Jr. "Calcium Absorption from Calcium Carbonate and a New Form of Calcium (CCM) in Healthy Male and Female Adolescents." *Am J Clin Nutr* (1988); 48: 1291–94.
20. Miller JZ, Smith DL, Flora L, Peacock M, Johnston CC Jr. "Calcium Absorption in Children Estimated from Single and Double Stable Calcium Isotope Techniques." *Clinica Chimica Acta* (1989); 183: 107–114.
21. Kanerva RL, Andon MB, Smith KT. "Bioavailability of Calcium from Supplemental and Food Fortification Sources." *FASEB J* (1989); 3: A771.
22. Kanerva RL, Andon MB. "Assessing Human Bioavailability Potentials of Calcium Sources Using a Rat Model." *J Bone Min Res* (1990); 5: S176.
23. Fox MM, Andon MB, Kanerva RL, Gulley BJ. "Impact of Saturated Fatty Acid Content of Plant Triglycerides on Calcium Bioavailability from CaCO3 and the CCM Calcium Delivery System." *FASEB J* (1990); 4: 1046.
24. Kanerva R, Luhrsen K, Andon MB, Smith KT, Mehansho H. "Calcium Bioavailability from Fruit Juices Fortified with CCM: Whole Body 47Ca Retention in Rats and Dogs." *J Bone Min Res* (1991); 6: S103.
25. Chatzidakis C, Kanerva RL, Andon MB, Smith KT. "Calcium Bioavailability from Various Sources Determined by Whole Body Versus Femur 47-Calcium Retention in Rats." *J Bone Min Res* (1992); 7: S273.

26. Andon MB, Lloyd T, Matkovic V. "Supplementation Trials with Calcium Citrate Malate: Evidence in Favor of Increasing the Calcium RDA During Childhood and Adolescence." *J Nutr* (1994); 124 (suppl.): 1412S–17S.
27. Dawson-Hughes B, Dallal GE, Krall EA, Sadowski L, Sahyoun N, Tannenbaum S. "A Controlled Trial of the Effect of Calcium Supplementation on Bone Density in Postmenopausal women." *N Engl J Med* (1990); 323: 878–83.
28. Dawson-Hughes B, Dallal GE, Krall EA, Harris S, Sokoll LJ, Falconer G. "Effect of Vitamin D Supplementation on Wintertime and Overall Bone Loss in Healthy Postmenopausal Women." *Annals Intern Med* (1991); 115: 505–12.
29. Johnston CC Jr, Miller JZ, Slemenda CW, Reister TK, Hui S, Christian JC, Peacock M. "Calcium Supplementation and Increases in Bone Mineral Density in Children." *N Engl J Med* (1992); 327: 82–87.
30. Lloyd T, Andon MB, Rollings N, et al. "Calcium Supplementation and Bone Mineral Density in Adolescent Girls." *JAMA* (1993); 270: 841–44.
31. Strause L, Saltman P, Smith KT, Bracker M, Andon MB. "Spinal Bone Loss in Postmenopausal Women Supplemented with Calcium and Trace Minerals." *J Nutr* (1994); 124: 1060–64.
32. Jackman LA, Millane SS, Martin BR, Wood OB, McCabe GP, Peacock M, Weaver CM. "Calcium Retention in Relation to Calcium Intake and Postmenarcheal Age in Adolescent Females." *Am J Clin Nutr* (1997); 66: 327–33.
33. Dawson-Hughes B, Harris SS, Krall EA, Dallal GE. "Effect of Calcium and Vitamin D Supplementation on Bone Density in Men and Women 65 Years of Age or Older." *N Engl J Med* (1997); 337: 670–76.
34. Lloyd T, Martel JK, Rollings N, Andon MB, et al. "The Effect of Calcium Supplementation and Tanner Stage on Bone Den-

sity, Content and Area in Teenage Women." *Osteoporosis Int* (1996); 6: 276–83.

35. Andon MB, Miller JZ, Slemenda CW, Johnston CC Jr, Smith KT. "Effect of Calcium Intake on Bone Mass in Children." *FASEB J* (1991); 5: 560.
36. Smith KT, Andon MB, Saltman P, Strause L. "Effects of Calcium (CCM) and Trace Mineral Supplementation on Bone Loss in Postmenopausal Women." *FASEB J* (1991); 5: 560.
37. Lloyd T, Andon MB, Rollings N, et al. "Effect of Calcium Supplementation on Total Body Bone Mineral Density in Adolescent Females." *J Bone Min Res* (1992); 7: S136.
38. Matkovic V, Jelic T, Warlaw G, Ilich JZ, Goel PK, Wright JK, Andon MB, Smith KT, Heaney RP. "Timing of Peak Bone Mass in Caucasian Females and Its Implication for the Prevention of Osteoporosis." *J Clin Invest* (1994); 93: 799–808.
39. *Physician's Resource Manual on Osteoporosis: A Decision Making Guide, 2nd ed.* (Washington, DC: National Osteoporosis Foundation, 1991).
40. National Research Council. *Recommended Dietary Allowances, 10th ed.* (Washington, DC: National Academy Press, 1989).

Chapter Two

1. Andon MB, Peacock M, Kanerva RL, De Castro JAS (1996).
2. Smith KT, Heaney RP, Flora L, Hinders SM (1987).
3. Miller JZ, Smith DL, Flora L, Slemenda C, Jiang X, Johnston CC Jr (1988).
4. Miller JZ, Smith DL, Flora L, Peacock M, Johnston CC Jr (1989).
5. Heaney RP, Weaver CM, Recker RR (1988).
6. NIH Consensus Development Panel on Optimal Calcium Intake (1994).

7. Recker RR, Bammi A, Barger-Lux J, Heaney RP. "Calcium Absorbability from Milk Products, an Imitation Milk, and Calcium Carbonate." *Am J Clin Nutr* (1988); 47: 93–95.
8. Sheikh MS, Santa Ana CA, Nicar MJ, Schiller LR, Fordtran JS. "Gastrointestinal Absorption of Calcium from Milk and Calcium Salts." *N Engl J Med* (1987); 317: 532–36.
9. Weaver CM, Plawecki KL (1994).
10. Heaney RP, Recker RR, Weaver CM. "Absorbability of Calcium Sources: The Limited Role of Solubility." *Calcif Tissue Int* (1990); 46: 300–04.
11. Recker RR. "Calcium Absorption and Achlorhydria." *N Engl J Med* (1985); 313: 70–73.
12. Food and Nutrition Board, Institute of Medicine (1997).
13. Wilson JW, Wilkinson-Enns C, Goldman JD, Tippett KS, Mickle SJ, Cleveland LE, Chahil PS (1997).
14. United States Department of Agriculture, Human Nutrition Information Service (1976–1989).
15. Heaney RP, Weaver CM, Fitzsimmons ML. "Influence of Calcium Load on Absorption Fraction." *J Bone Miner Res* (1990); 11: 1135–38.

Chapter Three

1. Matkovic V, Klisovic D, Ilich JZ. "Epidemiology of Fractures During Growth and Aging." In *Physical Medicine and Rehabilitation Clinics of North America: Osteoporosis,* ed. GH Kraft, V Matkovic (Philadelphia: W.B. Saunders Co., 1995), 415–40.
2. Food and Nutrition Board, Institute of Medicine (1997).
3. Johnston CC Jr, Melton LJ, Lindsay R, Eddy DM (1989).
4. Matkovic V, Jelic T, Warlaw G, Ilich JZ, Goel PK, Wright JK, Andon MB, Smith KT, Heaney RP (1994).
5. Nordin BEC, Chatterton BE, Need AG, Horowitz M. "The Definition, Diagnosis, and Classification of Osteoporosis." In

Physical Medicine and Rehabilitation Clinics of North America: Osteoporosis, ed. GH Kraft, V Matkovic (Philadelphia: W.B. Saunders Co., 1995), 395–414.

6. Matkovic V, Ciganovic M, Tominac C, et al. "Osteoporosis and Epidemiology of Fractures in Croatia. An International Comparison." *Henry Ford Hosp Med J* (1980); 28: 116–26.
7. Diamond TH, Thornley SW, Sekel R, Smerdely P. "Hip Fractures in Elderly Men: Prognostic Factors and Outcomes." *Med J Aust* (1997); 167: 412–15.
8. Zimmerman SI, Fox KM, Magaziner J. "Psychosocial Aspects of Osteoporosis." In *Physical Medicine and Rehabilitation Clinics of North America: Osteoporosis,* ed. GH Kraft, V Matkovic (Philadelphia: W.B. Saunders Co., 1995), 441–54.
9. Cook DJ, Guyatt GH, Adachi JD, et al. "Quality of Life Issues in Women with Vertebral Fractures Due to Osteoporosis." *Arthritis Rheum* (1993); 36: 750–56.
10. Roberto KA. "Women with Osteoporosis: The Role of the Family and Service Community." *Gerontologist* (1988); 28: 224–28.
11. Matkovic V, Fontana D, Tominac C, et al. "Factors Which Influence Peak Bone Mass Formation: A Study of Calcium Balance and the Inheritance of Bone Mass in Adolescent Females." *Am J Clin Nutr* (1990); 52: 878–88.
12. Seeman E, Hopper JL, Bach LA, Cooper ME, Parkinson E, McKay J, Jerums G. "Reduced Bone Mass in Daughters of Women with Osteoporosis." *N Engl J Med* (1989); 320: 554–58.
13. Johnston CC Jr, Slemenda CW. "The Relative Importance of Nutrition Compared to Genetic Factors in the Development of Bone Mass." In *Nutritional Aspects of Osteoporosis,* ed. P Burckhardt, RP Heaney (New York: Raven Press, 1992), 21–26.
14. Slemenda CW, Christian JC, Reed T, Reister TK, Williams CJ, Johnston CC Jr. "Long-Term Bone Loss in Men: Effects of Genetic and Environmental Factors." *Ann Intern Med* (1992); 117: 286–291.

15. Kelly PJ, Morrison NA, Sambrook PN, Nguyen TV, Eisman JA. "Genetic Influences on Bone Density and Bone Turnover." In *Physical Medicine and Rehabilitation Clinics of North America: Osteoporosis,* ed. GH Kraft, V Matkovic (Philadelphia: W.B. Saunders Co., 1995), 539–50.
16. Johnston CC Jr, Miller JZ, Slemenda CW, Reister TK, Hui S, Christian JC, Peacock M (1992).
17. Andon MB, Miller JZ, Slemenda CW, Johnston CC Jr, Smith KT (1991).
18. Peacock M, Johnston CC Jr, Miller JZ, Smith DL, Andon MB. "Calcium Supplementation in Children Decreases Calcium Absorption and Bone Turnover." *J Bone Min Res* (1991); 6: S271.
19. Peacock M, Andon MB, Kanerva R, Johnston CC Jr, Schuster C, Miller J, Smith D, Smith K. "Effect of Calcium Supplementation on Bone Accretion, Bone Turnover, Calcium Absorption Efficiency, and Iron Status in Children." *FASEB J* (1992); 6: A1957.
20. Hangartner TN. "Osteoporosis Due to Disuse." In *Physical Medicine and Rehabilitation Clinics of North America: Osteoporosis,* ed. GH Kraft, V Matkovic (Philadelphia: W.B. Saunders Co., 1995), 579–94.
21. Dalsky GP, Stocke KS, Eshani AA, Slatopolshy E, Lee WC, Birge SJ. "Weight-Bearing Exercise Training and Lumbar Bone Mineral Content in Postmenopausal Women." *Ann Intern Med* (1988); 108: 824–28.
22. Drinkwater BL. "Weight-Bearing Exercise and Bone Mass." In *Physical Medicine and Rehabilitation Clinics of North America: Osteoporosis,* ed. GH Kraft, V Matkovic (Philadelphia: W.B. Saunders Co., 1995), 567–78.
23. Huddleston AL, Rockwell D, Kulund DN, Harrison RB. "Bone Mass in Lifetime Tennis Athletes." *JAMA* (1980); 244: 1107–09.
24. Haapasalo H, Kannus P, Sievanen H, Pasanen M, Uusi-Rasi K, Heininen A, Oja P, Vuori I. "Effect of Long-Term Unilateral

Activity on Bone Mineral Density of Female Junior Tennis Players." *J Bone Miner Res* (1998); 13: 310–19.

25. Slemenda CW, Johnston CC Jr. "High Intensity Activities in Young Women: Site Specific Bone Mass Effects Among Female Figure Skaters." *Bone Miner* (1993); 20: 125–32.
26. Prior JC, Vigna YM, Schechter MT, Burgess AE. "Spinal Bone Loss and Ovulatory Disturbances." *N Engl J Med* 1990; 323: 1221–27.
27. Heinrich CH, Going SC, Pamenter RW, Perry CD, Boyden TW, Lohman TG. "Bone Mineral Content of Cyclically Menstruating Female Resistance and Endurance Trained Athletes." *Med Sci Sports Exercise* (1990); 22: 558–63.
28. Bilanin JE, Blanchard MS, Rusek-Cohen E. "Lower Vertebral Bone Density in Male Long Distance Runners." *Med Sci Sports Exerc* (1989); 21: 66–70.
29. Ormerod SD, MacDougall C, Webber J, et al. "The Relationship Between Weekly Mileage and Bone Density in Male Runners." *Med Sci Sports Exerc* (1990); 22: S62.
30. Myburgh K, Hutchins J, Fatarr AB, et al. "Low Bone Density As an Etiological Factor for Stress Fractures in Athletes." *Ann Intern Med* (1990); 113: 754–59.
31. Lloyd T, Triantafyllou ST, Baker ER, et al. "Women Athletes with Menstrual Irregularity Have Increased Musculoskeletal Injuries." *Med Sci Sports Exerc* (1986); 18: 374–79.
32. Shirreffs SM, Maughan RJ. "Whole Body Sweat Collections in Humans: An Improved Method with Preliminary Data on Electrolyte Content." *J Appl Physiol* (1997); 82: 336–41.
33. Valimaki MJ, Karkkainen M, Lamberg-Allardt C, Laitinen K, Alhava E, Heikkinen J, Impivaara O, Makela P, Palmgren J, Seppanen R. "Exercise, Smoking, and Calcium Intake During Adolescence and Early Adulthood As Determinants of Peak Bone Mass: Cardiovascular Risk in Young Finns Study Group." *Br Med J* (1994); 309: 230–35.

34. Vogel JM, Davis JW, Nomura A, Wasnich RD, Ross PD. "The Effects of Smoking on Bone Mass and Rates of Bone Loss Among Elderly Japanese-American Men." *J Bone Miner Res* (1997); 12: 1495–1501.
35. Kiel DP, Zhang Y, Hannan MT, Anderson JJ, Baron JA, Felson DT. "The Effect of Smoking at Different Life Stages on Bone Mineral Density in Elderly Men and Women." *Osteoporosis Int* (1996); 6: 240–48.
36. Hutchinson TA, Polansky SM, Feinstein AR. "Post-Menopausal Oestrogens Protect Against Fractures of Hip and Distal Radius." *Lancet* (1979); 2: 705–09.
37. Matkovic V, Ilich JZ, Andon MB, Hsieh LC, Tzagournis MA, Lagger BJ, Goel PK. "Urinary Calcium, Sodium, and Bone Mass in Young Females." *Am J Clin Nutr* (1995); 62: 417–25.
38. Massey LK, Whiting SJ. "Dietary Salt, Urinary Calcium, and Bone Loss." *J Bone Miner Res* (1996); 11: 731–36.
39. National Research Council (1989).
40. Devine A, Criddle RA, Dick IM, Kerr DA, Prince RL. "A Longitudinal Study of the Effect of Sodium and Calcium Intakes on Regional Bone Density in Postmenopausal Women." *Am J Clin Nutr* (1995); 62: 740–45.
41. Delmi M, Rapin CH, Bengoa JM, Delmas PD, Vasey H, Bonjour JP. "Dietary Supplementation in Elderly Patients with Fractured Neck of the Femur." *Lancet* (1990); 335: 1013–16.
42. Heaney RP. "Nutritional Factors in Osteoporosis." In *Annual Review of Nutrition,* ed. RE Olsen, DM Bier, DB McCormick (Palo Alto, CA: Annual Reviews Inc, 1993), 287–316.
43. Recker RR, Davies KM, Hinders SM, Heaney RP, Stegman MR, Kimmel DB. "Bone Gain in Young Adult Women." *JAMA* (1992); 268: 2403–08.
44. Wilson JW, Wilkinson-Enns C, Goldman JD, Tippett KS, Mickle SJ, Cleveland LE, Chahil PS (1997).

45. Lloyd T, Rollings NR, Eggli DF, Kiesekhorst K, Chinchilli VM. "Dietary Caffeine Intake and Bone Status of Postmenopausal Women." *Am J Clin Nutr* (1997); 65: 1826–30.
46. Cauley JA, Seeley DG, Ensrud K, Ettinger B, Black D, Cummings SR. "Estrogen Replacement Therapy and Fractures in Older Women." *Ann Intern Med* (1995); 122: 9–16.
47. Heaney RP. "Nutritional Factors in Bone Health in Elderly Subjects: Methodological and Contextual Problems." *Am J Clin Nutr* (1989); 50: 1182–89.
48. Colditz GA, Hankinson SE, Hunter DJ, Willet WC, Manson JE, Stampfer MJ, Hennekens C, Rosner B, Speizer FE. "The Use of Estrogens and Progestins and the Risk of Breast Cancer in Postmenopausal Women." *N Engl J Med* (1995); 332: 1589–93.
49. Nieves JW, Komar L, Cosman F, Lindsay R. "Calcium Potentiates the Effect of Estrogen and Calcitonin on Bone Mass: Review and Analysis." *Am J Clin Nutr* (1998); 67: 18–24.
50. NIH Consensus Development Panel on Optimal Calcium Intake (1994).

Chapter Four

1. Miller JZ, Smith DL, Flora L, Slemenda C, Jiang X, Johnston CC Jr (1988).
2. Miller JZ, Smith DL, Flora L, Peacock M, Johnston CC Jr (1989).
3. Johnston CC Jr, Miller JZ, Slemenda CW, Reister TK, Hui S, Christian JC, Peacock M (1992).
4. NIH Consensus Development Panel on Optimal Calcium Intake (1994).
5. Food and Nutrition Board, Institute of Medicine (1997).
6. National Research Council (1989).
7. Matkovic V, Jelic T, Warlaw G, Ilich JZ, Goel PK, Wright JK, Andon MB, Smith KT, Heaney RP (1994).

8. Andon MB, Kanerva RL, Schulte MC, Smith KT. "Effect of Age, Calcium Source, and Radiolabeling Method on Whole Body 47Ca Retention in the Rat." *Am J Physiol* (1993); 265 (Endocrino Metab 28): E544–48.
9. Sheikh MS, Santa Ana CA, Nicar MJ, Schiller LR, Fordtran JS (1987).
10. Recker RR, Bammi A, Barger-Lux J, Heaney RP (1988).
11. Smith KT, Heaney RP, Flora L, Hinders SM (1987).
12. Abrams SA, Grusak MA, Stuff J. "Calcium and Magnesium Absorption from Vegetables and Milk in Children." *FASEB J* (1997); 11: A573.
13. Heaney RP, Weaver CM, Recker RR (1988).
14. Dawson-Hughes B, Harris SS, Krall EA, Dallal GE (1997).
15. Johnston CC Jr, Slemenda CW(1992).
16. Matkovic V, Kostial K, Simonovic I, Buzina R, Brodarec A, Nordin BEC. "Bone Status and Fracture Rates in Two Regions of Yugoslavia." *Am J Clin Nutr* (1979); 32: 540–49.
17. Matkovic V, Ilich JZ. "Calcium Requirements for Growth: Are Current Recommendations Adequate?" *Nutr Rev* (1993); 51: 171–80.
18. Hu J-F, Zhao X-H, Jia J-B, Parpia B, Campbell TC. "Dietary Calcium and Bone Density Among Middle-Aged and Elderly Women in China." *Am J Clin Nutr* (1993); 58: 219–27.
19. Sandler RB, Slemenda C, LaPorte RE, Cauley JA, Schramm MM, Barresi ML, Kriska AM. "Postmenopausal Bone Density and Milk Consumption in Childhood and Adolescence." *Am J Clin Nutr* (1985); 42: 270–74.
20. Halioua L, Anderson JJB. "Lifetime Calcium Intake and Physical Activity Habits: Independent and Combined Effects on the Radial Bone of Healthy Premenopasual Caucasian Women." *Am J Clin Nutr* (1989); 49: 534–41.
21. Andon MB, Lloyd T, Matkovic V (1994).
22. Lloyd T, Andon MB, Rollings N, et al., (1993).

23. Teegarden D, Weaver CM. "Calcium Supplementation Increases Bone Density in Adolescent Girls." *Nutr Rev* (1995); 52: 171–73.
24. Jackman LA, Millane SS, Martin BR, Wood OB, McCabe GP, Peacock M, Weaver CM (1997).
25. Andon MB, Miller JZ, Slemenda CW, Johnston CC Jr, Smith KT (1991).
26. Peacock M, Johnston CC Jr, Miller JZ, Smith DL, Andon MB (1991).
27. Peacock M, Andon MB, Kanerva R, Johnston CC Jr, Schuster C, Miller J, Smith D, Smith K (1992).
28. Lloyd T, Rollings N, Andon MB, et al. "Determinants of Bone Density and the Effect of Calcium Supplementation in Young Women." *Third Bath Conference on Osteoporosis and Bone Measurements* (Bath, UK: 1992).
29. Lloyd T, Andon MB, Rollings N, et al (1992).
30. Lloyd T, Andon MB, Rollings N, et al. "Endogenous Estrogen Levels Modify the Effect of Calcium Supplementation on Bone Acquisition in Adolescent Girls." *J Bone Min Res* (1993); 8: S122.
31. Lloyd T, Andon M, Rollings, N, et al. "A Controlled Trial of Calcium Supplementation and Bone Density in Adolescent Females." *FASEB J* (1993); 7: A68.
32. Ilich JZ, Landoll JD, Andon MB, Matkovic V. "Calcium Metabolism During Puberty: A Longitudinal Study." *J Bone Min Res* (1995); 10: S464.
33. Lloyd T, Rollings N, Chinchilli V, Martel J, Eggli D, Demers LM, Andon MB. "The Effect of Starting Calcium Supplementation at Age 12 or 14 on Bone Acquisition in Teenage Girls." *J Bone Min Res* (1995); 10: S152.
34. Matkovic V, Hsieh L, Andon MB, Ilich JZ. "Skeletal Calcium Accretion as Determined by Balance Technique and Dual Energy X-Ray Absorptiometry." *J Bone Min Res* (1993); 8: S253.

35. Lloyd T, Martel JK, Rollings N, Andon MB, et al (1996).
36. Wilson JW, Wilkinson-Enns C, Goldman JD, Tippett KS, Mickle SJ, Cleveland LE, Chahil PS (1997).
37. Matkovic V, Klisovic D, Ilich JZ (1995).
38. Buhr AJ, Cooke AM. "Fracture Patterns." *Lancet* (1959); 1: 531–36.
39. Garraway WM, Stauffer RN, Kurland LT, et al. "Limb Fractures in a Defined Population. I. Frequency and Distribution." *Mayo Clin Proc* (1979); 54: 701–07.
40. Landin LA. "Fracture Patterns in Children." *Acta Orthop Scand* (1983); 54: 5S–95S.
41. Bailey DA, Wedge JH, McCulloch RG, et al. "Epidemiology of Fractures of the Distal End of the Radius in Children As Associated with Growth." *J Bone Joint Surg* (1989); 8: 125–30.

Chapter Five

1. Dawson-Hughes B, Dallal GE, Krall EA, Sadowski L, Sahyoun N, Tannenbaum S (1990).
2. Dawson-Hughes B, Dallal GE, Krall EA, Harris S, Sokoll LJ, Falconer G (1991).
3. Strause L, Saltman P, Smith KT, Bracker M, Andon MB (1994).
4. Smith KT, Andon MB, Saltman P, Strause L (1991).
5. Strause L, Saltman P, Smith KT, Andon MB. "Calcium, Copper, Manganese, and Zinc Supplementation Sustains Spinal Bone Density in Postmenopausal Women." *J Bone Min Res* (1991); 6: S282.
6. Dawson-Hughes B, Harris SS, Krall EA, Dallal GE (1997).
7. Department of Health and Human Services. *Surgeon General's Report on Nutrition and Health.* (Washington, DC: U.S. Government Printing Office, 1988) [DHHS publication (PHS) No. 88 50210].

8. Nilas L, Christiansen C, Rodbro P. "Calcium Supplementation and Postmenopausal Bone Loss." *Br Med J* (1984); 289: 1103–06.
9. Ettinger B, Genant HK, Cann CE. "Postmenopausal Bone Loss Is Prevented by Treatment with Low-Dosage Estrogen with Calcium." *Ann Intern Med* (1987); 106: 40–45.
10. Riis B, Thomsen K, Christiansen C. "Does Calcium Supplementation Prevent Postmenopausal Loss?" *N Engl J Med* (1987); 316: 173–77.
11. Heaney RP (1989).
12. Heaney RP (1993).
13. Sheikh MS, Santa Ana CA, Nicar MJ, Schiller LR, Fordtran JS (1987).
14. Andon MB, Peacock M, Kanerva RL, De Castro JAS (1996).
15. Smith KT, Heaney RP, Flora L, Hinders SM (1987).
16. Miller JZ, Smith DL, Flora L, Slemenda C, Jiang X, Johnston CC Jr (1988).
17. Miller JZ, Smith DL, Flora L, Peacock M, Johnston CC Jr (1989).
18. Kanerva RL, Andon MB, Smith KT (1989).
19. Peacock M, Andon MB, Stegner J, Decastro J. "Bioavailability of Calcium from CCM-Fortified Apple Juice and Orange Juice." *J Bone Min Res* (1991); 6: S161.
20. Cumming RG. "Calcium Intake and Bone Mass: A Quantitative Review of the Evidence." *Calcif Tissue Int* (1990); 47: 194–201.
21. National Research Council (1989).
22. Strause L, Saltman P, Smith K, Andon M. "Trace Elements and Bone Metabolism." In *Nutritional Aspects of Osteoporosis,* ed. P Burckhardt, RP Heaney (New York: Raven Press, 1992), 223–33.
23. Wilson JW, Wilkinson-Enns C, Goldman JD, Tippett KS, Mickle SJ, Cleveland LE, Chahil PS (1997).
24. Pennington JAT, Young BE, Wilson DB. "Nutritional Elements in U.S. Diets: Results from the Total Diet Study, 1982–86." *J Am Diet Assoc* (1989); 89: 659–64.

25. Holick MF. "McCollum Award Lecture, 1994: Vitamin D—New Horizons for the 21st Century." *Am J Clin Nutr* (1994); 60: 619–30.
26. Food and Nutrition Board, Institute of Medicine (1997).
27. Holick MF, Shao Q, Liu WW, Chen TC. "The Vitamin D Content of Fortified Milk and Infant Formula." *N Engl J Med* (1992); 326: 1178–81.
28. Chen TC, Heath H, Holick MF. "An Update on the Vitamin D Content of Fortified Milk from the United States and Canada." *N Engl J Med* (1993); 329: 1507.
29. Orwoll ES, Oviatt SK, McClung MR, Deftos LJ, Sexton G. "The Rate of Bone Mineral Loss in Normal Men and the Effects of Calcium and Cholecalciferol Supplementation." *Ann Intern Med* (1990); 112: 29–34.
30. Lips P, Graafmans WC, Ooms ME, Bezemer PD, Bouter LM. "Vitamin D Supplementation and Fracture Incidence in Elderly Persons." *Ann Intern Med* (1996); 124: 400–06.
31. Chapuy MC, Arlot ME, Duboeuf F, et al. "Vitamin D3 and Calcium to Prevent Hip Fractures in Elderly Women." *N Engl J Med* (1992); 327: 1637–42.
32. Ricci TA, Chowdhury HA, Heymsfield SB, Stahl T, Pierson RN Jr, Shapses SA. "Calcium Supplementation Suppresses Bone Turnover During Weight Reduction in Postmenopausal Women." *J Bone Min Res* (1998); 13: 1045–50.

Chapter Six

1. NIH Consensus Development Panel on Optimal Calcium Intake (1994).
2. Food and Nutrition Board, Institute of Medicine (1997).
3. Whiting SJ. "The Inhibitory Effect of Dietary Calcium on Iron Bioavailability: A Cause for Concern?" *Nutr Rev* 1995; 53: 77–80.

4. Whiting SJ, Wood RJ. "Adverse Effects of High-Calcium Diets in Humans." *Nutr Rev* (1997); 55: 1–9.
5. Andon MB, Ilich JZ, Tzagournis MA, Matkovic V. "Magnesium Balance in Adolescent Females Consuming a Low- or High-Calcium Diet." *Am J Clin Nutr* (1996); 63: 950–53.
6. Deehr MS, Dallal GE, Smith KT, Taulbee JD, Dawson-Hughes B. "Effects of Different Calcium Sources on Iron Absorption in Postmenopausal Women." *Am J Clin Nutr* (1990); 51: 95–99.
7. McKenna AA, Ilich JZ, Andon MB, Wang C, Matkovic V. "Zinc Balance in Adolescent Females Consuming a Low- or High-Calcium Diet." *Am J Clin Nutr* (1997); 65: 1460–64.
8. Ilich JZ, McKenna AA, Badenhop NE, Clairmont A, Andon MB, Nahhas RW, Matkovic V. "Iron Status, Menarche, and Calcium Supplementation in Young Females." (In press).
9. Matkovic V, Ilich JZ, Hsieh L, Tominac C, Tzagouris M, Luhrsen KR, Smith KT, Andon MB. "Calcium, Magnesium, and Zinc Balances in Females During Early Puberty." *J Bone Min Res* (1993); 8: S152.
10. Curhan GC, Willett WC, Rimm EB, Stampfer MJ. "A Prospective Study of Dietary Calcium and Other Nutrients and the Risk of Symptomatic Kidney Stones." *N Engl J Med* (1993); 328: 833–38.
11. Lemann J. "Composition of the Diet and Calcium Kidney Stones." *N Engl J Med* (1993); 328: 880–82.
12. Curhan GC, Willett WC, Speizer FE, Spiegelman D, Stampfer MJ. "Comparison of Dietary Calcium and Supplemental Calcium and Other Nutrients As Factors Affecting the Risk of Kidney Stones in Women." *Ann Intern Med* (1997); 126: 497–504.
13. United States Department of Agriculture, Human Nutrition Information Service (1976–1989).
14. Liebman M, Chai W. "Effect of Dietary Calcium on Urinary Oxalate Excretion After Oxalate Loads." *Am J Clin Nutr* (1997); 65: 1453–59.

15. Coe FL, Parks JH, Webb DR. "Stone-Forming Potential of Milk or Calcium-Fortified Orange Juice in Idiopathic Hypercalciuric Adults." *Kidney Int* (1992); 41: 139–42.
16. Denke MA, Fox MM, Schulte MC. "Short-Term Dietary Calcium Fortification Increases Fecal Saturated Fat Content and Reduces Serum Lipids in Men." *J Nutr* (1993); 123: 1047–53.
17. Wilson JW, Wilkinson-Enns C, Goldman JD, Tippett KS, Mickle SJ, Cleveland LE, Chahil PS (1997).
18. Heaney RP, Smith KT, Recker RR. "Meal Effects on Calcium Absorption." *Am J Clin Nutr* (1989); 49: 372–76.
19. Recker RR (1985).
20. Strause L, Saltman P, Smith K, Andon M (1992).
21. Strause L, Saltman P, Smith KT, Bracker M, Andon MB (1994).
22. National Research Council (1989).
23. Argiratos V, Samman S. "The Effect of Calcium Carbonate and Calcium Citrate on the Absorption of Zinc in Healthy Female Subjects." *European J Clin Nutr* (1994); 48: 198–204.
24. Wood RJ, Zhang JJ. "High Dietary Calcium Intakes Reduce Zinc Absorption and Balance in Humans." *Am J Clin Nutr* (1997); 65: 1803–09.
25. Whiting S. "Safety of Some Calcium Supplements Questioned." *Nutr Rev* (1994); 52: 95–105.

Chapter Seven

1. National Institutes of Health. *Fifth Report of the Joint National Committee on Detection, Evaluation, and Treatment of High Blood Pressure.* (NIH Publication No. 93–1088, 1993).
2. Department of Health and Human Services (1988).
3. McCarron DA, Morris CD, Young E, Roullet C, Drueke T. "Dietary Calcium and Blood Pressure: Modifying Factors in Specific Populations." *Am J Clin Nutr* (1991); 54: 215S–19S.

4. Hamet P. "The Evaluation of the Scientific Evidence for a Relationship Between Calcium and Hypertension," ed. D Raiten. *J Nutr* (1995); 125 (suppl. 2S): 311S–400S.
5. Hung J-S, Huang T-Y, Wu D, Yen M-F, Tsai S-H, Dahl HP, Neaton J, Dahl JC. "The Impact of Dietary Sodium, Potassium and Calcium on Blood Pressure." *J Formosan Med Assoc* (1990); 89: 17–22.
6. Trevisan DM, Krogh V, Farinaro E, Panico S, Mancini M. "Calcium-Rich Foods and Blood Pressure: Findings from the Italian National Research Council Study (the Nine Communities Study)." *Am J Epidemiol* (1988); 127: 1155–63.
7. Iso H, Terao A, Kitamura A, Sato S, Naito Y, Kiyama M, et al. "Calcium Intake and Blood Pressure in Seven Japanese Populations." *Am J Epidemiol* (1991); 133: 776–83.
8. Criqui MH, Langer RD, Reed DM. "Dietary Alcohol, Calcium, and Potassium: Independent and Combined Effects on Blood Pressure." *Circulation* (1989); 80: 609–14.
9. Gruchow HW, Sobocinski KA, Barboiak JJ. "Calcium Intake and the Relationship of Dietary Sodium and Potassium to Blood Pressure." *Am J Clin Nutr* (1988); 48: 1463–70.
10. Anonymous. "The Effects of Nonpharmacologic Interventions on Blood Pressure of Persons with High Normal Levels—Results of the Trials of Hypertension Prevention, Phase I." *J Am Med Assoc* (1992); 267: 1213–20.
11. Zoccali C, Mallamaci F, Delfino D. "Double-Blind Randomized, Crossover Trial of Calcium Supplementation in Essential Hypertension." *J Hypertens* (1988); 6: 451–55.
12. Nowson C, Morgan T. "Effect of Calcium Carbonate on Blood Pressure in Normotensive and Hypertensive People." *Hypertension* (1989); 13: 630–39.
13. Bierenbaum ML, Wolf E, Bisgeier G, Maginnis WP. "Dietary Calcium—A Method of Lowering Blood Pressure." *Am J Hypertens* (1988); 1: 149S–52S.

14. Kynast-Gales SA, Massey LK. "Effects of Dietary Calcium from Dairy Products on Ambulatory Blood Pressure in Hypertensive Men." *J Am Diet Assoc* (1992); 92: 1497–1501.
15. Allender PS, Cutler JA, Follman D, Cappuccio FP, Pryer J, Elliott P. "Dietary Calcium and Blood Pressure: A Meta-Analysis of Randomized Clinical Trials." *Ann Intern Med* (1996); 124: 825–31.
16. Saito K, Sano H, Furuta Y, Fukuzaki H. "Effect of Oral Calcium on Blood Pressure Response in Salt-Loaded Borderline Hypertensive Patients." *Hypertension* (1989); 13: 219–26.
17. Rich GM, McCullough M, Olmedo A, Malarick C, Moore TJ. "Blood Pressure and Renal Blood Flow Responses to Dietary Calcium and Sodium Intake in Humans." *Am J Hypertens* (1991); 4: 642S–45S.
18. Belizn JM, Villar J, Zalazar A, Rojas L, Chan D, Bryce GF. "Preliminary Evidence of the Effect of Calcium Supplementation on Blood Pressure in Normal Pregnant Women." *Am J Obstet Gynecol* (1983); 146: 175–80.
19. Lopez-Jaramillo P, Narvaez M, Weigel RM, Yepez R. "Calcium Supplementation Reduces Risk of Pregnancy-Induced Hypertension in an Andes Population." *Br J Obstet Gynaecol* (1989); 96: 648–55.
20. Lopez-Jaramillo P, Narvaez M, Felix C, Lopez A. "Dietary Calcium Supplementation and Prevention of Pregnancy Hypertension." *Lancet* (1990); 335: 293.
21. Belizn JM, Villar J, Gonzalez L, Campodonico L, Bergel E. "Calcium Supplementation to Prevent Hypertensive Disorders of Pregnancy." *N Engl J Med* (1991); 325: 1399–1405.
22. Levine RJ, Hauth JC, Curet LB, Sibai BM, Catalano PM, Morris CD, DerSimonian R, Esterlitz JR, Raymond EG, Bild DE, Clemens JD, Cutler JA. "Trial of Calcium to Prevent Preeclampsia." *New Engl J Med* (1997); 337: 69–76.

23. Gillman MW, Hood MY, Moore LL, Nguyen UDT, Singer MR, Andon MB. "Effect of Calcium Supplementation on Blood Pressure in Children." *J Pediatr* (1995); 127: 186–92.
24. Richter F, Newmark HL, Richter A, Leung D, Lipkin M. "Inhibition of Western-Diet Induced Hyperproliferation and Hyperplasia in Mouse Colon by Two Sources of Calcium." *Carcinogenesis* (Oxford, 1995); 16: 2685–89.
25. Garland CF, Garland FC, Gorham ED. "Can Colon Cancer Incidence and Death Rates Be Reduced with Calcium and Vitamin D?" *Am J Clin Nutr* (1991); 54: 193S–201S.
26. Slattery ML, Sorenson AW, Ford MH. "Dietary Calcium Intake As a Mitigating Factor in Colon Cancer." *Am J Epidemiol* (1988); 128: 504–14.
27. Garland CF, Shekelle RB, Barrett-Connor E, et al. "Dietary Calcium and Vitamin D and Risk of Colorectal Cancer: A 19-Year Prospective Study in Men." *Lancet* (1985); 1: 307–09.
28. Lipkin M. "Application of Intermediate Biomarkers to Studies of Cancer Prevention in the Gastrointestinal Tract: Introductions and Perspective." *Am J Clin Nutr* (1991); 54: 188S–92S.
29. Lipkin M, Newmark HL. "Effect of Added Dietary Calcium on Colonic Epithelial Cell Proliferation in Subjects at High Risk for Familial Colon Cancer." *N Engl J Med* (1985); 313: 1381–84.
30. Wargovich MJ, Lynch PM, Levin B. "Modulating Effects of Calcium in Animal Models of Colon Carcinogenesis and Short-Term Studies in Subjects at Increased Risk for Colon Cancer." *Am J Clin Nutr* (1991); 54: 202S–05S.
31. National Research Council (1989).
32. Denke MA, Fox MM, Schulte MC (1993).
33. Davidson MH, Maki KC, Kong JC, Dugan LD, Torri SA, Hall HA, et al. "Long-Term Effects of Consuming Foods Containing Psyllium Seed Husk on Serum Lipids in Subjects with Hypercholsterolemia." *Am J Clin Nutr* (1998); 67: 367–76.

34. Davidson MH, Dugan LD, Burns JH, Bova J, Story K, Drenan KB. "The Hypocholesterolemic Effects of Beta-Glucan in Oatmeal and Oat Bran. A Dose-Controlled Study." *JAMA* (1991); 265: 1833–39.

Chapter Eight

1. United States Department of Agriculture, Human Nutrition Information Service (1976–1989).
2. Food and Nutrition Board, Institute of Medicine (1997).
3. Wilson JW, Wilkinson-Enns C, Goldman JD, Tippett KS, Mickle SJ, Cleveland LE, Chahil PS (1997).
4. Weaver CM, Heaney RP, Martin BR, Fitzsimmons ML. "Extrinsic vs. Intrinsic Labeling of the Calcium in Whole-Wheat Flour." *Am J Clin Nutr* (1992); 55: 452–54.
5. Heaney RP, Recker RR, Weaver CM (1990).
6. Weaver CM, Plawecki KL (1994).
7. Heaney RP, Weaver CM, Recker RR (1988).
8. Abrams SA, Grusak MA, Stuff J (1997).
9. Recker RR, Bammi A, Barger-Lux J, Heaney RP (1988).
10. Smith KT, Heaney RP, Flora L, Hinders SM (1987).
11. Sheikh MS, Santa Ana CA, Nicar MJ, Schiller LR, Fordtran JS (1987).
12. Andon MB, Peacock M, Kanerva RL, De Castro JAS (1996).
13. Miller JZ, Smith DL, Flora L, Slemenda C, Jiang X, Johnston CC Jr (1988).
14. Miller JZ, Smith DL, Flora L, Peacock M, Johnston CC Jr (1989).
15. Cleveland LE, Cook AJ, Wilson JW, Firday JE, Ho JW, Chahil PS. "Pyramid Servings Data: Results from the USDA's 1994 Continuing Survey of Food Intake by Individuals." U.S. Department of Agriculture, Agricultural Research Service, Beltsville Human Nutrition Research Center, Food Surveys' Research Group (Riverdale, MD: 1997).

INDEX

INDEX